It Could Happen to You

GERALD H THORNHILL

This book is a work of nonfiction.

Ordering Information:

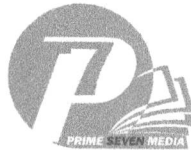

Prime Seven Media
518 Landmann St.
Tomah City, WI 54660

Printed in the United States of America

This book is dedicated to Mr Neil Smith,
Consultant General and Colorectal Surgeon of East Surrey
Hospital, whom I have come to look upon as a friend.
And to my bother Cyril, who has been a friend,
and the best I could wish for.

Table of Contents

Fifty percent of us in the UK will be diagnosed with cancer. That awful statistic means it is highly likely all of us are affected one way or another. We know someone who had it, got it, or died from it.

The author was told he had bowel cancer in August 2018 and was operated on by the surgeon Neil Smith at East Surrey Hospital on August 23rd. The cancerous part of his bowel was removed, he recovered, and life returned to normal.

Until 16th May 2019.

This is the ongoing story of the cancer he has had, and still has, the NHS, and how the disease has affected him and those around him

CHAPTER ONE

2018
A routine blood test

I have been lucky in life as far as my health is concerned. I can count on one hand the times I have been ill. Seriously ill, that is. I don't mean colds and flu and the minor maladies we all get from time to time—I mean illness that was serious enough to be admitted to a hospital.

At the age of eleven, a lump appeared on the left side of my neck. It was big, "the size of a golf ball," I heard one doctor describe it. I endured a great deal of barracking from fellow schoolchildren. "Ooh, don't come near me, Thornhill, that thing on your neck could be catching," and similar such remarks—some quite nasty. Children can be very cruel to one another.

We lived in Felixstowe at the time, and Mum took me to see Dr Pool our local GP. He decided I needed to have my tonsils removed and this was carried out at the Borough General Hospital in Ipswich, and my adenoids were removed at the same time.

The lump remained. So, it was back to Dr Pool, who then decided it was my teeth and arranged for the school dentist to remove several at the back of my mouth. This was accomplished.

The lump remained.

Mum decided it was time for a second opinion.

As we walked into his surgery Dr Read looked up and said, "Good god, Mother. That boy should be in hospital!" And he picked up the phone.

It was the winter of 1947, and the next day, Mum and I walked up the hill through the slush and snow to the East Suffolk and Ipswich Hospital to see a specialist, Mr McKenzie. Mr McKenzie was the ear nose and throat specialist and very much of his time. By that I mean he behaved and seemed to believe he was someone special and those around him all inferior.

"Undo your shirt, boy." He ordered in a sharp and intimidating tone.

I undid three or four buttons at the top of the shirt and he shouted. "Good god, boy, that's no good. Undo it all. I need to listen to your chest. How do you expect me to do it like that!"

He examined my chest and neck carefully, and eventually told Mum I had a TB infected gland, and it would have to be drained, and so a few days later, I was in the hospital, operated on, and the gland drained. A few weeks later the lump re-appeared, and

I was back in hospital for another operation, this time to remove the infected gland. This was accomplished, and I had no further trouble in that area.

The only other time I have been ill enough for a hospital stay was during my time in the RAF. I contracted scarlet fever and was taken into the isolation ward of the camp hospital where I slept for about 36 hours, and on wakening, found myself fit and well.

* * *

A year or so before I entered the RAF, I started smoking. One of the greatest mistakes I have ever made—and there have been innumerable—but smoking is probably the biggest and the one I regret the most. There were several reasons for taking up this objectionable habit: peer pressure as most of my friends smoked. Films, particularly Hollywood films with people like Humphrey Bogart in them. I thought smoking would make me appear cool and sophisticated, urbane, and grown-up. It probably did none of these things, but it did make me poorer than I needed to be and caused me to smell of cigarettes for most of the time, and in later life, as we shall see, created major problems. Several times, I tried to give the habit up to save money and many times in the mid 50s after a report was published blaming cigarettes for lung cancer. During my time in the RAF, cigarettes were sold in the NAAFI extremely cheaply, so by the time I came home I was well hooked, and it wasn't until I was forty that I became so annoyed the tobacco companies had me hooked I was able, when offered a cigarette to say, "No thanks. I've given them up."

For the next fifty years, I enjoyed good health. During that time, I met and married Heather. She was seventeen; I was ten years older. Heather had a sunny personality, always smiling. To her the glass was always half full; never ever half empty, she continually looked on the bright side and always saw the best in people. I would say to new friends and acquaintances, "You must meet my wife, you'll like her," knowing with great certainty that they would. They always did. Heather was just plain likeable.

We married in 1968 and moved into an old, thatched cottage in Stansted, not far from her parents' house. The next few years were spent renovating the place with a lot of help from Heather's dad. Heather, on leaving school, had worked at Caton's the village supermarket, but after our marriage obtained a job with Co-Op Travel and worked on their ticket desk at Stansted Airport checking in the passengers. I had left the coach company I had been working for and, with the help of her dad, Charlie, had obtained a job with the BAA in the MT section at the airport. After a few years, I was promoted into the Operations Department, a more interesting area of airport work—runway inspections, bird scaring, marshalling, runway lighting checks, and innumerable other tasks all connected with maintaining the safety of the aircraft as they manoeuvred around the airfield.

Heather and I got along together well. Never rowed, we did argue occasionally, but disagreements were rare, and when we did, she would end it by switching on her captivating smile and saying something like, "Well, never mind, Tott, it's possible we could both be wrong. Let's dance!" And she would put her arms around me, and we would dance a few steps around the kitchen as I hummed 'The Cuckoo Waltz', Heather giggling, me laughing; the argument forgotten. She called me 'Tott', I never found out why. Short for totter? I would totter a little after too many pints which I have to admit occurred more often than it should have, so was that the reason?

I called her 'Bumble' because she could never settle on anything for long. Like a bumble bee moving from one flower to another. Heather would move from one task in the house to another, never settling for long on anything. She had a low boredom threshold. She was good with people, had a knack of getting on with everyone. Complete strangers, friends, relatives, it didn't matter. She had talent for putting them at ease and making them relax. It was a gift I admired, an ability I have never achieved. We were married but as the years rolled by, we became the very best of friends too and that is the best kind of marriage, isn't it?

We didn't have children. Heather wasn't keen, and I wasn't bothered one way or the other. I wasn't enthusiastic, I think because I had been influenced by couple's I knew who had children and I had observed the worry, cost, anxiety, and sheer hard work that seemed to accompany the appearance of them. Not to mention the responsibilities that go with having a family. I think Heather was a little frightened about the idea of giving birth. She certainly never displayed any maternal instinct, but I must admit we never discussed having a family in depth. We should have. There are so many things we should have talked about and didn't. An omission I bitterly regret. It's very strange, but recently, now the end of my life is in sight, I keep thinking maybe we should have thought seriously about having children. I am certain Heather would have been a good mother. She had the right personality for it, the right temperament. Would I have been a good father? Not so sure about that. I think I'm too much like *my* father to be able to say yes to that question.

I won't pretend the relationship between Heather and I was a perfect one without any kind of trouble because, of course, it wasn't. But there is no doubt in my mind that the few occasions of disharmony and short periods of unhappiness we did have were always resolved by the inbuilt skill Heather had with people and her perpetual optimism.

In 1993, my younger brother's 25-year marriage to Pat was heading for the rocks. Their marriage had produced two children, Stephen and Lyndsay. He was an HGV driver, and at this time was working for a double-glazing company, *Twin Windows*, delivering to various places in England. If his deliveries brought him to the Stansted area, which it often did, he would call in to see us at out cottage on the edge of the village, which we encouraged him to do and would invite him along to social events we attended and also the various airport parties that were organised most weekends. As the months went by and his visits more regular, it became increasingly clear his return home to his now unhappy marriage was with some reluctance.

They divorced and put their house in Stockport on the market, agreeing to split the proceeds. Cyril started to look for somewhere to live. He continued to visit us, often coming down by train and staying weekends.

After one of his weekend visits, Heather said to me, "Why don't you ask your brother if he would like to live with us permanently?"

I said, "Are you sure? It might not work. You know—the three of us together all the time, sharing the house."

"On the other hand, it might, and I think it would. We all get on well, don't we?"

It was true, we did. Heather had a mischievous sense of humour which I knew appealed to Cyril as much as me, and I had always got on well with Cyril. I had tried to help him in the early days of his marriage which had got off to a bad start due, I think, to the early arrival of Stephen, not being able to afford to buy a house, and consequently was forced to move in with my Mum, who was not the easiest of people to live with.

That weekend, I invited him out for a drink and put the idea to him. I could tell straightaway the suggestion appealed. Cyril is not the type to rush into anything without carefully examining the subject first. He was all for the proposal but suggested we try it for six months. "Or a year if you like," he said, "and after a year assess it and decide if we should continue. If not, we go our separate ways with no hard feelings."

"We should share all the expenses," I said. "The rates, water, electricity and all that kind of thing. And we'll go through it all with Heather when we get home."

The idea worked. And it worked well. We shared everything. The three of us enjoyed life together for almost thirty years.

In 1973, I was promoted and transferred to Gatwick. We moved to the village of Bolney in West Sussex and found an old cottage that required work. It was in the hands of a receiver and after some negotiations we, were able to get it for an excellent price. Heather obtained a job with British Caledonian Airways in their offices in Crawley and later Staff Travel at Gatwick, and later still, was transferred to British Airways. When Be-Cal was taken over by BA she became one of BAs employees.

Because one of the perks working for an airline is cheap travel, we began to travel ourselves. We visited America, Canada, South Africa, Brazil, Mexico, Hong Kong, Mainland China, and many other areas of the world. Because she worked in Staff Travel and most of the BA staff visited that office, Heather was often recognised when we were jetting off somewhere, and, because in this life it is not what you know but who you know, there were many occasions when we were moved from the cheap seats in the back into business class at the front. When this kind of thing happened, she would dig me in the ribs and say, "Aren't you glad you met me, Tott?"

Our travels together were delightful times and have left me with many happy memories.

I never regretted marrying Heather. She overlooked my faults, was loyal, supportive, forgiving, and had infinite patience with me. She looked after me so well—she would even make phone calls for me as she knew I became frustrated and annoyed when put on hold and forced to listen to music for minutes on end. She brought me much happiness, never failed to encourage any of my enthusiasms.

Every year, she would make an appointment at our local surgery for me to have a blood test. "But I'm fine." I would say.

"A blood test will confirm that, won't it?" She would answer. And it always did.

Until five years ago.

CHAPTER TWO

A little Anaemic

TUESDAY 22ND MAY

I was in with Dr Richardson waiting for her to tell me the result of my recent blood test. She was fiddling with the mouse and staring at the screen. On my past half-dozen or more visits to get the result of blood tests, the doctor had done the same and usually said something like, "Yes, everything seems fine, kidneys, liver, everything looks fine, and you look fine." But this time, I could sense a difference as she continued to move the mouse around and stare at the screen.

I said, "What's up?" More for something to say than believing there was something up. She didn't answer and continued to stare at the screen. There was a silence. From the waiting room, I heard a voice call out a name, the scrape of a chair and footsteps.

Dr Richardson nodded at the screen and said, "Well, Mr Thornhill, it's telling me you are a little anaemic."

"Anaemic? What does that mean?'

"It means your haemoglobin is low. You are lacking red blood cells. We must find out why."

"But I feel fine."

"Yes, you do look well, but we must find out the cause of this anaemia. I'll arrange for you to have an ultrasound at St Vic's and…" She pulled out a plastic tube from a cupboard and handed it to me, "I'll need a stool sample, okay?"

"Yes, of course, but I'm going to America in a couple of weeks."

"I'll tell the hospital it's urgent, and with a bit of luck, they will arrange for you to have it before you go, okay?"

Four days later, a phone call from Queen Victoria Hospital: Could I come for a scan on Friday?

It was impressively quick.

FRIDAY 4TH MAY

Heather is with me, and we go via Lingfield to drop off the stool sample at the surgery on the way to Queen Vic's. Queen Victoria Hospital in East Grinstead is famous for the care of World War Two pilots who suffered horrific burns during their battle for Britain and does wonderful work for burn victims today. It has the atmosphere of the late 1940s -1950s. I'm not sure why. Maybe it's the temporary look of the buildings; maybe it's the general feel of the place. It reminds me of cottage hospitals as they used to be.

It's a pay and display car park. £2 and hour (not like cottage hospitals as they used to be.) It's full, so we sit in the car waiting for a space to appear, and eventually, one does. "How long do you think we will be here?" I say to Heather.

She shrugs her shoulders. "Couple of hours?"

I shell out £4. We are not late, and soon a nurse invited me into an examination room.

"The toilet is just down the corridor to your left," she informs me.

"Oh, okay." I say. There is a short silence. "Why are you telling me that?" I ask.

"I need you to empty your bladder," she says.

"Oh, right." I act as instructed and I'm soon lying on a bunk-like bed half undressed and being ultra sounded. It is much like pregnant women have when checking the baby. The nurse stares at the screen as she moves the device over my stomach and chest and asks me to move on to my side. She studies the screen. The procedure only takes a few minutes.

"Can't see anything wrong," she says eventually. "I'll send a report to your doctor."

Heather and I walk back to the car park. "I hope that's the last of me visiting hospitals." I say to her.

"Yes, let's hope so, but if not well, it will be for your own good, won't it?"

"Yeah, I suppose so."

WEDNESDAY 9TH MAY 2018

Back in the surgery to see Dr Richardson and get the results of the tests. I asked Heather to come with me again so she can ask questions I don't think of.

After a short period of sitting in the waiting room reading a three-month-old Sussex Life (Heather) and two-month-old Peoples Friend (me), we watch Dr Richardson peer at the computer screen. The analysis of the stool sample had not been received from the lab, and we discussed whether I should submit another sample but decided the delay is due to the early May Bank Holiday, and the result will probably come through in a day or two.

WEDNESDAY 16ᵗʰMAY 201

I heard nothing from the surgery so as had been arranged for weeks, I flew out to join my brother, Cyril, at our place in Florida. He had left the UK three weeks before, and we planned to spend another six weeks there. During that time, Heather would join us. He met me at Fort Lauderdale Airport. An American neighbour, Dennis, had brought him down in his car, and we drive north to Stuart, where we have a two-bed-flat, or condominium, on a marina called Circle Bay that sits on the side of the wide St Lucie River.

It was a warm evening and in spite of it being such a long day—getting up at 7 AM, a ten hour flight and a one-and-a-half hour road journey plus a five hour time change, I was not too tired to sit on the lanai in the warm evening air watching the boats sale past and have a beer with my little brother before going to bed.

"How did the blood test go?" Cyril asked me.

"Fine," I said without thinking and then realized it wasn't fine. "No—not fine," I correct. "Apparently, the tests have shown I'm a little anaemic."

"What? You don't look anaemic."

"How do you look when you are anaemic?"

"Pale, you know, ill looking."

"I think it's mild, though, I don't really know. The doctor arranged a couple of tests. I'll get the results when I get home."

"But that's not until the middle of June."

"Well, the surgery will ring Heather if the doctor wants to see me before then." I took a sip of beer and shrugged my shoulders. "As I said, I think it's mild. I'll probably have to take iron tablets or something."

On the river a large yacht sailed past. We both watched it. They are having a party on board. Through the warm evening air, laughter and music float across the water.

SATURDAY 19ᵀᵗʰMAY 2018

The temperature has been in the eighties with blue skies and wispy clouds in the mornings, but thunderstorms in the afternoons; though, we have been able to get on the Brompton's and cycle down to "The Sailors Return"—our favourite bar. We have also been along to the Friday evening party on the deck and met neighbours and friends and chatted, swopped stories, told jokes, translated: "No, no, a fag is a cigarette!"

As usual, we were greeted with great enthusiasm: "Hey Gerry, great to see you again… "Welcome back, you are looking younger than ever, how do you do it? And "Waddya doin here, the wedding's tomorrow!"

It's weird how Royalist so many Americans are. Everyone I have spoken to seem to be excited about the Royal Wedding of Prince

Harry and Megan, yet the country fought a revolutionary war in the 1770s to get rid of all things royal. I suppose the new princess, the Duchess of Sussex (I doubt she has ever been to Sussex) is American and has a lot to do with the present royal hysteria.

We were both up early. CBS, NBC, ABC and Fox—all the main TV channels were full of the wedding. They are encamped at Windsor. The weather there seemed suitably royal, bright, sunny, and warm. I made tea while C slotted bread into the toaster. We sat and watched the wedding. The pomp. The circumstance. There was a happy clappy choir, and American Evangelist, Bishop Michael Curry who delivered a fiery sermon that lasted for 15 minutes or so. He waved his arms about; it was not the type of thing or he the type of person St George's Chapel would be used to hearing. A two second shot of the Queen and Prince Phillip showed them both looking stony-faced. Clearly not impressed with the bishop's performance.

"How long do you give it?" C asked me as the happy couple walked down the aisle.

"Five years, ten at the most." I said.

"I doubt it will last that long," he answered. She'll get fed up with all the protocol and disciplines of the palace, the bowing and scraping. And she'll want to visit her friends in the US and take any children they have. The controllers in the palace won't like that. Part of the Royal family running around free in America? No way!"

Cynical, both we were, I think.

I phoned Heather. She had been filling in for Cyril on his 107 Meridian FM radio show and I have woken myself up a couple of times to listen to her. She did a good job, and it's been strange listening to her so far away yet seeming so close. We chat for a while. "Everything okay?" "What's the weather like?" "Did you watch the wedding?"

After a few minutes, Heather said, "The surgery rang."

There is a fluttering in my stomach. "Oh?"

"The doctor wants to see you. I told them you were abroad and wouldn't be back until June 20th. The girls said you should make an appointment as soon as you are back."

"Did she say why the doctor wants to see me?"

"I didn't ask—she wouldn't have told me, anyway, and I doubt if she knows."

"Should I get a flight back, do you think?"

"I think you should ring the surgery on Monday and see if you can talk to Dr Richardson."

"Okay," I said, "I'll do that."

I put the phone down. Cyril said, "What's up? You look worried."

I told him, "The doctor wants to see me. I'll bet something has come up with those tests."

"It may be nothing. You worry too much. Let's get on the bikes and go down to Flanagan's and have something to eat."

"Yeah, and something to drink."

CHAPTER THREE

"I would like you to see a specialist".

TUESDAY 22ND MAY 2018

I phoned the surgery yesterday.

"Dr Richardson is with a patient; I can't interrupt her." The receptionist said.

"She wants to see me, apparently, but I'm in Florida, if I could just have a quick word to see if it's anything urgent. If it is I'll come back, but if not, well, I don't come back to the UK until June 20th.

"I understand. I can arrange a time for you to call her. Can you ring us back tomorrow?"

I got up early this morning and called the surgery again. A different receptionist answers. I explain it all again.

"I spoke to your colleague yesterday, she was going to arrange a time for me to speak to the doctor," I tell her.

She puts me on hold.

It's another sunny morning. A clear blue sky, I look through the sliding glass doors. Out on the river a speedboat is towing a young lad on water skis at a fast rate of knots. They whizz past a slow-moving yacht, its sails flapping. Not much wind, I conclude. The weatherman on TV this morning told us there will be more rain this afternoon. No going out on the bikes today.

"Hello, Mr Thornhill?"

"Yes, hello."

"Dr Richardson will speak to you now."

There is a clunk, a silence, and another clunk. "Mr Thornhill, I believe you are in Florida—lucky you!"

"Hello, Dr Richardson. I understand you want to see me. I planned to be out here until June 20th. Should I come back?"

"That's for you to decide. I would like you to see a specialist, it's possible you may have to have a colonoscopy to help find out what the problem is. Perhaps you could have one out there?"

What the hell's a colonoscopy?

I think quickly. The medical insurance I have is limited. Knowing insurance companies, I'll bet somewhere in the small print there will be a clause excluding 'investigative medical problems. I could probably arrange to have a colonoscopy here but knowing how the American health system works, I am confident it would cost a small fortune.

"I think I should come back," I say.

"Well, Mr Thornhill, you can go on holiday at any time, but if you return, I can get you an appointment with a specialist within a fortnight." Dr Richardson answers.

"Okay, I'll come back."

I tell Cyril, "I've got to go back. Sorry, you'll be on your own again."

"Don't worry. You are doing the right thing. We'll have to get on to Norwegian Air. When are you thinking of going?"

"As soon as I can get a flight."

We get on to Norwegian Air and the only flight they can offer is from Orlando on May 31st arriving home June 1st. There is nothing from Fort Lauderdale and, of course, because I have changed the return date there is a cost, £400. The fact I have already paid for a return flight cuts no ice with them. I've changed the date, and that's enough to screw more money out of me.

There has been a great deal of rain during my stay at Circle Bay this time, much more than I have experienced before. I haven't had the chance to laze about by the pool like I usually do, but we have been able to get out on the bikes a few times and, of course it has been very warm with the temperature in the high eighties.

We usually go out with our neighbours, Chuck, and Laurie, though, I shouldn't describe them as neighbours. Over the years, they have become good friends. We always spend at least one evening with them when we are here; out for a meal or something, but Laurie hasn't been well and with hospital visits a night out together hasn't been possible this time.

"You're going home, Gerry? You've only just got here!" It's not out of choice, I tell them and explain as best I can. "You are doing the right thing," they both assure me.

This evening we have been able to meet up with Steve Campbell— another good American friend—he is, or should I say was, a realtor, or estate agent, and is the man who found us our place at Circle Bay in 2002. We all meet at Ruby Tuesdays in Palm City, Mary and Dennis, more friends are also there. I explain again why I am going home so soon.

"Don't you have long waiting lists, you know, if it's something serious you could die waiting. Isn't that true?"

"That's' what Trump wants you to believe," I say, and all of a sudden, I'm defensive about the NHS. "No, it's not true. If you have something life threatening, you are dealt with very quickly. Our National Health Service has its faults, of course, it has, but if it came to a choice between your system, based on profits for the insurance companies and the medical and pharmaceutical industry—I'll take ours any time."

"Huh, Trump," said Steve disparagingly, that man should be taken out and shot. He's a disgrace." The conversation moves on to Trump and his presidency, and it soon becomes clear he is not particularly popular amongst most of those present.

THURSDAY 31ST/ FRIDAY 1ST OF JUNE

Our friend Adele, another neighbour who we have known now for several years, has given us a set of her car keys and as she always does when we are here and told us to use it whenever we want. How generous some Americans can be. Adele is up in New York visiting her son, so now we are speeding north toward Orlando in her Toyota Varris on Interstate 95, sitting in light coloured leather seats, radio playing, *"You are listening to one-oh-three-point seven the only golden oldies station on the Treasure Coast".* The Beatles come on *"She's Leaving Home."* Such a good song.

Cyril drops me outside No 2 terminal.

"I'll get parked and join you in a few minutes to make sure you get away." With my bag, I get into Norwegian Air's Upper-Class queue. A few minutes go by. The check-in gets busy. "Next please!"

Then I see Cs head of white hair pushing through the crowds. He looks panicky.

"What's up?" I ask.

"Have you got the car keys? It's one of those key-less cars. You only need the key in your pocket to start it or for it to unlock. It's still where I dropped you, and they are threatening to tow it away. I've been given three minutes." He taps his pockets. "I haven't got them so I can't start it."

I remember I moved the car at Circle Bay nearer to the condo when we were getting ready to leave. I feel in my pockets, find them, hand them over."

"Thank goodness!" He dashes off and is back in ten minutes looking much more relaxed. The short queue moves forward, and I'm soon checked in.

"Let us know you get home okay," he says.

"Course I will. Don't go off with any strange women and behave yourself, remember, I won't be here to look after you."

He gives me a hug—this is unusual—hugging is something alien to us both.

"I'll ignore that," he says. Love to Heather."

It was a night flight, and I was able to sleep for two or three hours.

Heather meets me at Gatwick with a bright smile and a warm hug. This one not so alien.

As we drive along, she tells me a letter has arrived informing me an appointment has been made to see a specialist, Mr Smith, at East Surrey Hospital next Wednesday morning. I look out of the window; everything is very green, and it's warm and sunny. A good-to-be-alive-day. It can't be anything serious, can it? I feel fine, no different to how I felt a year ago—five years ago. I get tired these days, but as I keep reminding myself, I'm getting on a bit and old people do get tired, don't they? It's natural. This specialist, Mr Smith, will probably put me on a course of tablets, or something like that, and that will fix it. No more concerns.

"… you're not, are you?" Heather has been talking. I've not been listening.

"Sorry, love, what did you say?"

"I said you are not worrying, are you? Because you shouldn't, they are looking into it. They'll sort it out whatever it is. Dr Richardson is being thorough and arranging all this for you. That's good, isn't it?"

"Yes, 'course it is. I'm not worrying."

Well, not too much.

CHAPTER FOUR

The Specialist

WEDNESDAY 6TH JUNE

Heather and I drive down to East Surrey Hospital in Redhill. It is still warm and sunny, and we get parked without difficulty at £2 and hour. After reporting to the outpatient's desk, we are directed to a waiting room where we sit for a half-hour, then I am called forward to be weighed and a few minutes after the weigh-in we are ushered into the presence of the specialist.

He sits at a desk but stands as Heather and I enter the room and holds out his hand grasping mine warmly and shaking it and then Heather's with equal warmth. A nurse stands in the background smiling. My fears that this was going to be like meeting the arrogant, unsympathetic, Mr McKenzie at the Ipswich and East Suffolk Hospital all those years ago are dispelled. This chap exudes friendliness, and we are both immediately comfortable with him.

"Mr and Mrs Thornhill, do sit down. I'm Neil Smith, call me Neil," he says. A junior doctor is sitting in the corner. He is introduced and he smiles as he shakes our hands. We sit. Mr Smith—Neil—studies the computer screen. "Now," he says, looking at us both, "tell me why you think you are here."

This takes me aback. Shouldn't he know why we are here? But I go through it: A routine annual blood test… Dr Richardson telling me I am a little anaemic telling me we must find out why… stool sample… her arranging this appointment today…

Neil listens intently until my description of events comes to a halt. "Right," he says, smiling. "The trouble is Lingfield Surgery don't always seem to get things right. They have sent your records over, but they are not complete. Maria will get on to them and have what we want sent over. So, if you don't mind waiting a little longer? As soon as we get them, we'll have you back in here and have another chat. Okay?"

We don't have to wait long before we are sitting at his desk again. More warm smiles. He has a way of relaxing me. Heather too, I think.

"Well, I'm sorry," he says. Looking like he means it. "But we still haven't got what we want from Lingfield. This is what I propose—we send you along for a blood test now. Maria will take you, and we need a stool sample; it can be taken to Crawley Hospital if that is easier for you and then we'll decide the way forward, so we'll be in touch in about a week. Is that okay with you?"

"Yes, of course. Fine." We stand, shake hands, and follow Maria to where I have the blood test.

* * *

I receive a letter from Mr Neil Smith to Dr Richardson, at Lingfield Surgery dated 6th June In it he says I may not need a colonoscopy. I'm pleased about that. Perhaps this whole thing is something and nothing after all. The anaemia of little consequence, a few iron tablets and back to normal. Is that how it is going to end up? But then I get another copy of a letter sent by Neil to Dr Richardson in which he says I *should* have one. I guess it was the result the blood test and stool sample that changed his mind.

So, I will have to have a colonoscopy. Not a pleasant prospect, but if it helps to sort this problem out...

SATURDAY 30TH JUNE

As instructed, we are at the Endoscopy Unit, East Surrey Hospital at 15.15. on the 30th of June. I've already drunk a couple of pints of water this morning, but a smiling nurse urges me to drink more. My temperature and blood pressure taken. I am questioned about my bowel movements. Cyril wanders off, and Heather sits with me. Eventually, I am ushered into the procedure room where the deed is to be done. I sign a consent form. The nurse asks me to remove my trousers and lie on a trolley. Mr Aslam, the consultant, introduces himself; the nurse inserts a cannula into the back of my hand through which a sedative will flow that should make me feel drowsy and, according to the paperwork, cause me not to remember too much about the whole thing.

Mr Aslam directs me to lie on my side with my knees slightly bent. The nurse positions a pulse monitoring probe on my index finger and a small tube supplying oxygen is inserted into my nostril. I am tense. I try to think of anything but what is actually happening. I try to imagine a sun-kissed Caribbean Island, the shore curving away, the sun warm on my face, in the bay two or three sailboats anchored in the crystal clear water, a few yards along the shoreline there is a bar, a crowd of people sitting by it drinking, enjoying…

It doesn't work. As Mr Aslam manoeuvres his instrument, I jump a couple of times, much to his irritation as twice he says, "You must relax." An instruction I found impossible to comply with.

The operation takes about thirty minutes. I can't say it was painful, just uncomfortable, and, well, intrusive. Obviously. The sedative, which was to relax me, make me feel drowsy and cause me to hardly remember any of it, fails to do any of those things.

"You should be pleased, they are being thorough," Heather tells me.

I can't argue with that, thorough is the word.

About ten days later, I'm sitting at home on my own. Heather has gone shopping, Cyril is at Meridian FMs studio for his usual Monday morning show, and I'm listening to him ranting on about the amount of rubbish in the streets of East Grinstead, one of his favourite gripes, when the phone rings. It's Maria, one of the Clinical Nurse Specialist's on Neil Smith's team, "Mr Thornhill? Mr Smith has asked me to speak to you. He would like you to have a Pet Scan, it is—" I interrupt her. "I had a scan a week or so ago."

"Yes, this is a different type. It will give us more information about your lung."

"My lung? I'm sorry Maria, what has my lung got to do with the problem with my bowel?"

There is a short silence broken by a hum on the line, a door slams, then Maria says, "The scan you had the other week has shown up a small spot. It needs to be checked. It's just a precaution; it's possibly nothing. You'll get a letter from Guildford, okay?"

I say 'yes' and put the phone down and stare out of the window trying to take in what I have just heard.

Guildford? That's where you go if you've got cancer.

SATURDAY 28TH JULY

Heather and Cyril took me to Guildford. We found the scanning unit easily enough tucked away at the back of the hospital and was able to park close to the reception (for free!)

It must have been boring for them as the procedure took over two hours. After a 'tracer' was injected, I had to rest for an hour, then lay on a bed in the scanner room which moved me through the ring of the machine while I was instructed, "Hold your breath! Breathe normally... Hold your breath! Breath normally..."

The results are to be sent to Mr Smith.

CHAPTER FIVE

Verdict

WEDNESDAY 8TH AUGUST 2018

Another lovely warm and sunny day. Back to East Surrey this morning, accompanied by Heather, to see Mr Smith. He will now have studied the results of the various investigations and tests I have had over the last few weeks and, presumably, has decided what the problem is and what should be done about it.

This summer must be the best I can remember, it is even better than 1959. The sun is out again, and it is beautifully warm. It's one of those days when you feel good to be alive. We are not kept waiting too long before we are ushered into Mr Neil Smith's office. Big welcoming smile. "Mr and Mrs Thornhill, good to see you again. Do sit down."

Once again, we are both struck by his friendly charm. Perhaps East Surrey Hospital runs a Charm School for their specialists.

We sit down and both smile at Maria, the specialist nurse sitting nearby. Neil studies the computer screen for a couple of minutes and then says, "Well, Mr Thornhill, we have had a report of the CAT-scan that you had on your chest," he swings the computer screen toward us, "there was a place there," he points to the scanned image of my chest, on the screen, "that we thought might be a problem, but we are assured by the chest experts that it's nothing, so…" he smiles, "that's good enough for me."

"I had a chest infection earlier this year," I say, "maybe that had something to do with it?"

He tells me I need surgery on my bowel which is what is causing the anaemia. He picks up a booklet and turns to one of the pages and pointing to a coloured diagram of the bowel begins to explain about the surgery he says I need. I hear words like 'right hemicolectomy' and 'anastomotic leak' and, although Neil is carefully explaining it all to me, I'm not grasping his words at all because as he is speaking he hands me a couple of booklets and some leaflets and I glance down at them taking in the titles:

'A Guide to Colorectal CANCER "Help With The Cost Of CANCER,' 'Supporting You Through CANCER "We're Here For You—Macmillan CANCER Support."

The word is leaping off the pages at me. Neil's voice has faded off.

Heather has been asking questions. I've not been listening. She takes my hand in hers, "Are you all right, Tott?" I don't answer. I can't answer. It feels like something is squeezing my insides. I have a sudden empty, sick-like feeling. My throat has gone dry.

Neil says, "If you go with Maria, she will take you somewhere quiet and answer any of your questions and I'll see you on the 23rd, okay?"

We all stand, I manage to say, "Yes, okay," as we shake hands. Heather and I follow Maria out of the room, along a corridor and into a small office. Maria is talking to me, but I'm not sure what she is saying.

I didn't expect this. I should have, it was never going to be just a prescription for iron tablets, of course, it wasn't.

Maria says, "This kind of news is distressing, Mr Thornhill, I understand." She can see I am shocked. She talks to us, her words are kind and sympathetic, understanding, and compassionate. I'm still unable to speak; there is a big lump in my throat, and I'm frightened if I attempt to say anything I will break down. And then, to my dismay, a tear rolls down my face. This is ridiculous, I need to pull myself together, I quickly wipe my eyes, but they have both seen it. Heather leans across and grasps my hand tightly. Maria says, "We've caught it early—you will get over it. I promise." I nod and try to smile, but the word is still bouncing around in my head.

Cancer. I've got Cancer. Cancer is fatal. You get cancer. You die. For Christ's sake, what's going on here? I feel fine. Am I going to die? Well, we all die, but, honestly, I'm not ready for that yet.

Heather has been talking to Maria, she turns to me, "Is that okay with you, Tott?'

"What? Sorry." My voice sounds strangled. "Is what okay?"

"Maria is going to take you to the pre-admission clinic. If you go there today, it saves us a journey. Otherwise, we'll have to come back next week. I'll meet you at the coffee shop when you've finished, all right?"

I nod, stand, and follow Maria out of the room and down to the pre-admission clinic. It's a long walk down a wide corridor, past the Purple Zone, through the Orange Zone, the Green Zone. Patients in wheelchairs ride by, a middle-aged woman on crutches catches my eye and smiles as she hobbles past; a porter pushing a trolley containing an unconscious elderly man goes by. We pass a garden area where patients, relatives, and friends are sitting in the bright sunshine chatting. I try to make small talk with Maria, but my voice still sounds quivery, and we reach the pre-admission clinic in silence. I am given a form containing four or five pages of questions all to do with my mental and physical health; I am filling it out when Maria leaves me saying, "Don't hesitate to call me if you have any questions or if there is anything I can help you with." She smiles, touches my hand, "Are you all right?"

I try to smile back, fail.

I am taken into another room where a blood sample is taken, then an electrocardiograph and MRSA screening. My blood pressure is taken and the nurse taking it notices my swollen ankles. I tell her it's a side effect of the blood pressure tablets I take. She calls in an older, more senior nurse who studies my ankles and asks, "What tablets do you take?"

"Amlodipine." I tell her.

She pulls a face and shakes her head. "Come into my office, would you, Mr Thornhill?"

She waves me into a chair. "My name is Chris. Are you on your own?" I tell her 'no' my wife is in the coffee lounge. "Well, we need her here," she says, "What's her name?" I tell her and she turns to her colleague and says, "Do you mind?"

I am now becoming concerned. Is there something else? "Is there something wrong?" I ask, but she has picked the phone up and is tapping out numbers. I hear the ringtone. She says to me, "All these surgeries use Amlodipine," she shakes her head in disapproval, and then, "Hello, Neil? I have Mr Thornhill with me… yes…he's taking Amlodipine and it's… five… yes… he's scheduled for the 23rd …"

The conversation continues for another minute or so and ends with Chris saying, "Yes, I agree, that's good, okay." She puts the phone down and turns back to me, "Right, Mr Thornhill, it will be okay. We will have to see about putting you on to something else when you are with us."

She has an air of efficiency and gives me the impression she is the type that won't put up with any nonsense. "Is there anything wrong?" I ask again, "I mean apart from what I've got wrong?"

She shakes her head. "No, no, it's just that I'm not keen on Amlodipine, there are better alternatives, but it seems to be prescribed, well, too often in my opinion."

The younger nurse returns with Heather. Introductions are made.

"I wanted you together because I need to go through this with you both so that nothing comes as surprise," the senior nurse tells us.

The next fifteen minutes are taken up with her explaining, in some detail, what I should expect to experience during my four- to-six-day stay in the hospital, which starts on August 23rd. I should prepare myself physically, walk, cycle; eat a well-balanced diet… I am to have Laparoscopic (Keyhole) surgery, which means performing surgery with the use of a fibre optic camera and specialised surgical instruments introduced into the abdomen through 1cm incisions.

She talks about complications that could occur: Blood clots could develop due to lack of movement. I will be given white stockings to wear and injections of Heparin, a drug used to thin the blood, and I'll be encouraged to move around early in my recovery; leakage at the join (anastomosis of the bowel) is also a complication but only occurs in less than 5% of patients. So that's all right, then.

Hopefully.

After the operation, I will go into the high dependency unit for a while, and I'll have several tubes attached to me when I awake: an intravenous drip to give me the fluids I will need; a catheter and an epidural supplying painkillers.

I will be in East Surrey Hospital between four and seven days and full recovery will take up to three months.

Chris asks if we have any questions and tells us if between now and my admission on the 23rd I am concerned about anything we should contact one of the specialist nurses attached to Neil Smith's team.

As we walk back down the long corridor, Heather asks me if I want to get a coffee or tea before we drive home, but I say 'no,' my head is still in a kind of whirl; a jumble of incoherent thoughts. I've got cancer yet I feel fine, no different to how I felt this time last year, or the year before. Shouldn't I be feeling ill?

"What would happen if I didn't have this surgery? Did I ask that?" I ask Heather.

"Yes, you did. He said you would be okay for months, maybe years, but eventually it would get worse, and it could spread and... Why are you asking that, Tott?"

"I couldn't remember if I asked him what would happen if I didn't have it."

Over the next few days, I read the leaflets and booklets handed to me. Much of the information doesn't seem to apply, but I read it all anyway. I go to Google and look up some statistics and read: "Bowel cancer survival is improving and has more than doubled in the last 40 years." So that's good.

I read: "Seven in 10 people in England diagnosed with bowel cancer aged 15-39 survive their disease for five years or more, compared with 4 in 10 people diagnosed aged 80 and over.

Not so good.

I try to tell myself that after all, I am 81 so that's not a bad life. I know if I dropped dead today people would say, 'Well he had pretty good innings.' But this tactic doesn't work. These sorts of thoughts are no comfort whatsoever. The older I get the more enjoyable and the more precious life becomes. I want it to go on and on. Preferably without cancer.

CHAPTER SIX

Surgery

THURSDAY 23RD AUGUST 2018

It's warm and sunny again, a blue sky, warm breeze, the sort of day you want to go down to the beach, walk along the Downs, take a cycle ride, have a picnic, sit outside a country pub somewhere and sip a pint. Do anything except go into hospital.

Heather and I make our way to the Surgical Admissions Lounge at East Surrey Hospital. About a dozen people sit there, male and female. It's easy to work out who will be admitted and who are friends or relatives giving moral support. Those being admitted look the way I feel: apprehensive, worried, nervous, a little scared. They are probably having the same thoughts as me: will the operation be successful? Will the surgeon's knife slip?

Their ages range from forty-odd to one elderly guy who looks even older than me, though as you will see in a couple of seconds, I am wrong—he is younger. After a few minutes spent people studying, a nurse invites me into a side-room and takes my blood pressure, temperature, and oxygen level.

I return to the lounge and Mr Smith comes to see us. "I normally have my oldest patient in for surgery first," he tells us. "But although you are the oldest, we are seeing today, Mr Thornhill, you are also the fittest, so I'm afraid you will be the last. Sorry about that."

He turns to Heather. "We have your phone number, and I'll call you when I have some news, okay?"

I urge Heather to go home, as it is now obvious, I am going to be waiting here most of the day. She wishes me luck accompanied by one of her especially lovely smiles. She tells me to try not to worry and assures me everything is going to be all right.

I am handed a piece of paper and asked to sign. I do. Is this sealing my fate I wonder. It is the middle of the afternoon before a nurse comes in and asks me to confirm my name and date of birth, gives me a gown to wear, and I'm wheel-chaired to an anti-room near to the theatre, and I'm told to make myself comfortable on a bed. Although the long days wait has done nothing to lessen my apprehension, these last few minutes before I go under the knife become quite interesting, if not entertaining. I am waiting to be wheeled in for the surgery. There are three nurses in the room with me (one male, two female). They stand and sit by a desk about fifteen feet from where I lie answering the phone and filling out forms. One of them, a girl about twenty-five or so, starts to tell her colleagues about her father, who, she discovered when he died a few months previously, had fathered twenty-two children besides herself.

"What? By different women?" Her male colleague asks.

"Yes."

"You mean you've got twenty-two half brothers and sisters you didn't know you had?"

"Yes."

"How did you find out?" The other nurse asks.

"Well, when he died, several of them turned up at the funeral. Two were from New Guinea, three from someplace in Africa, and one from Australia." She laughs, "It was quite an interesting event."

"Good god!" The other female nurse exclaims. "I bet it was. Did your mother know?"

"Yes, apparently she did. The only one who showed any surprise or was in any way shocked was me."

"What did your dad do? I mean apart from…Well, travel the world and doing a lot of… travelling?"

"You'll never guess—he was—" The phone rings interrupting her.

"Hello? Mr Thornhill? Yes, yes, okay."

The male nurse comes over to me. "Okay, you are on, Mr Thornhill, I'm going to wheel you through. Are you okay?"

I'll never know what her dad did for a living now.

"Yes," I say and wonder if I am, and it's only now a familiar thought flits through my mind and then stops and backs up and settles for a minute or two: operations sometimes go wrong. I try to push away the picture this creates in my head, but it is stubborn and keeps creeping back. My heart rate, blood pressure, and oxygen levels are taken, and a cannula is inserted into my arm, and I'm asked if I'm okay and there are other questions directed at me which I can't remember and were clearly just to waste time while the anaesthetic takes effect. The anaesthetist's assistant asks my name and date of birth and now the anaesthetist is talking to me, and I'm trying to concentrate on his words. "You'll get a warm feeling in your bum, and after that, you won't feel too much," he says.

I look around for Mr Smith but can't see him. Has he forgotten me?

"Keep still, Mr Thornhill." The anaesthetist is leaning over me. "How's it going? Feel anything yet?"

"Not really," I say, and I'm beginning to worry that it may not be working. I remember reading a few weeks ago about a woman who woke up in the middle of an operation because her anaesthetist got it wrong. I look at his face for any sign of concern, but there is none, just a smile.

Before I can entertain more doubts, a pleasant warm feeling starts creeping into my backside and voices, faces, the lights, and then me all fade to black.

FRIDAY 24ᵀᴴ AUGUST

I can hear a noise. A machine is running. A nurse is looking down at me.

"Do you feel sick, Mr Thornhill?" I shake my head. "What is your date of birth?" she asks.

"Seventh of April nineteen…" I stop. My voice sounds weak, and my head feels fuzzy. My mind goes blank. For God's sake—what year was it? Then a feeling of relief, "Thirty-seven," I say.

She gives a slight nod and puts something in my ear. "I'm just taking your temperature, Mr Thornhill and then we need to check your blood pressure, okay?" I nod and realise there are tubes in my nose. Oxygen. I become aware other tubes are attached to me, a drip in a vein in my left arm and a catheter in my bladder.

"Do you have any pain?" she asks me.

I shake my head. "Well, a bit here." I touch my lower chest.

I notice a porter hovering by the foot of the bed. "We are going to take you down to the ward now," she says. "We'll give you something for the pain."

"Copthorne, right?" the porter says.

"Yes," the nurse answers.

Along a corridor, lights above my head sliding by, people walking past, the rattle of lift doors closing, the hum of machinery, lift doors opening, around a corner, around another corner. We enter a ward and slow down by the reception counter.

"Area 4 bed A," one of the nurses says.

CHAPTER SEVEN

Copthorne Ward

FRIDAY 24ᵀᴴ AUGUST

I can hear a noise, a rhythmic sound, not far from where I lie. There is a slight pain in my chest. The noise is some sort of machine next to the bed. A nurse is looking down at me. "Can you tell me your date of birth?" she asks. I tell her. "Do you have any pain?" I nod, touch my lower chest where the pain seems to be getting worse. The nurse puts something in my hand. "Press this button," she says, "if it gets too bad, and the pain will go. Is there anything you want?"

"Could I have a drink of orange?"

"Still orange, you can't have fizzy orange."

"That's fine." The pain is getting worse, so I press the button she has given me and now notice it is attached to one of two cannulas in my right arm. I try to pull myself up to look around, but it's too much of an effort. I feel weak and sore. The nurse returns and hands me a glass of orange with a straw and I suck greedily. "You should sleep," she says, "how is the pain?"

"It's nearly gone, that button is magic," I say, and she smiles and tells me to press it again if the pain returns and then points to another button hanging over the side of the bed and tells me to press it if I need help for any reason.

"I can't sleep like this," I tell her and try to turn on to my side, but the effort is too demanding.

"I'll help you," she says and leans down and helps me move onto my side. 'What is your name? "I ask.

"Kunju," she says.

I fall asleep again.

The pain is back; it wakes me. I press the magic button and stare up at the ceiling for a couple of minutes. The overhead lights are on. Above and to the side is a television on a movable bracket with a telephone next to it; on the wall behind my bed a whiteboard proclaims: "Gerald Thornhill" and "Soft." With an effort, I pull myself up and look around. There are four beds. The one next door is completely hidden by the curtains that are pulled around it.

An old boy opposite stares across in silence. In the left-hand corner, a younger man, fifty maybe, is sitting by his bed and looking out of the window. The man next to the old boy opposite is out of bed, dressed, and looks as if he is getting ready to go home, packing his hold-all, folding pyjama's and looking pleased.

I examine my stomach. A plaster covers my navel and there are two smaller plasters on either side. I still have drips attached to me, various plastic lines delivering nutrients, and the shots of morphine via the magic button and the catheter. The pain has faded away. I wonder if Neil Smith called Heather as he said he would.

I'm given a menu and asked to tick what I want for lunch and supper and told I can only have the foods marked with an "S". A male nurse comes in pushing a small green-coloured trolley with a large and a substantial looking door. Attached to the side is a typed notice:

"PLEASE DO NOT DISTURB THE NURSE GIVING OUT MEDICATION" and "PATIENT SAFETY IS ESSENTIAL WHEN ADMINISTERING DRUGS."

He stops by my bed and studies some paperwork and then says, "Good morning, Gerald." He is tall, dark, has a very slight accent; he is Asian, I guess.

"I have some pills for you, he says." He places a small plastic container on the wheeled table by my bed and a glass of water. Inside the plastic container are two pills, different colours.

"What are they for?" I ask.

"One is anti-sickness, the other a blood thinner."

"Okay. What's your name?"

"Mathew," he tells me. His English is impeccable. He pushes the cart across to the old boy opposite, "Good morning, James," he says and receives a grunt in reply.

I start to doze off again, but a nurse wakes me by taking my blood pressure, temperature, and oxygen level, but first asked me my date of birth, which this time I can recite without hesitation. I fall asleep.

I awake to a group of people at the foot of the bed staring down at me. Neil Smith and his team. "How do you feel?" he asks.

"Okay," I say and then pause thinking about it. "Yes, okay," I say again but more firmly this time.

He tells me the surgery went well, asks if I have felt sick, I tell him no, he asks if I have any pain and I tell him I did but it has faded off. He looks pleased and he and his group move off and over to the guy in the corner next to the window. I pick up my Kindle and start to read and after a while fall asleep again.

I wake up as lunch is being served. I get myself into a sitting position and manage to eat the filled baked potato, but not the tomato soup which tasted quite repellent, but it was compensated by the jelly and ice cream for sweet which was good. In the afternoon, I doze off again. The pain has faded, and I haven't needed to use the magic button at all.

I wake up to Heather's smiling face peering down at me. "Hello, how are you? Are you feeling okay?"

I try to gather my thoughts… Yes, bowel cancer…hospital… operation… Copthorne ward—it all floods back. "I keep falling asleep," I say.

She leans down and kisses me. "It's the anaesthetic. You look all right. Mr Smith called me, I didn't think he would, but he did— that was good of him, wasn't it? He said everything went well. Your brother is parking the car, he'll be here in a minute."

It's good to see her smiling face. She holds my hand, Cyril joins us, and we chat. I talk about the long wait in the Admissions Lounge yesterday and the food. There's a new family restaurant opened just up the road, Cyril tells me, and they are going to try it on the way home.

"Huh, it's all right for some," I say.

Heather pats my hand. "You'll soon be out of here, when do you think, Monday?"

"I don't see why not, I feel fine, though I haven't tried walking yet, and Monday is a Bank Holiday, do they release patients on a Bank Holiday?"

They leave after an hour or so and then supper is served. I'm not hungry but eat lemon sponge and custard and sip at the 'nourishing' drink they keep giving me. In the evening the chap in the corner by the window has visitors—his whole family by the look of it. There are five or six people round his bed, sitting, standing, talking, laughing, the radio is on tuned to the hospital's own station playing requests. The result, incongruously, is a noisy party atmosphere.

TUESDAY 28TH AUGUST

I wake with intense pain; it's early in the morning—one o'clock, two o'clock? The ward is quiet, lights out. My mind is filled with the agony of the pain in my chest, and I keep coughing, I can think of nothing else but the pain. I can hear someone moaning. I'm lying on my stomach and manage to push myself around and on to my back hoping this will help. The moaning continues, and I then realise it is me.

One of the booklets given to me mentioned something about 'effective pain control being an essential part of the Enhanced

Recovery Programme.' Okay, where is it? That's what I need, pain control. Right now. This minute.

I feel around for the emergency call button. I can't find it. It should be hanging on the side of the bed. It isn't. Should I shout the way James, opposite, often does? I'm getting desperate and feel around again. The bloody thing isn't here. For Christ's sake! I pull myself up and try to peer over the side of the bed and then I feel it under my leg, the cable has got itself wrapped around my waist. I get hold of it, press the button, and hold it pressed for several seconds. This is urgent, please hurry. A minute passes, it seems like an hour. Another minute, another hour, and yet another.

At last, she's here. She switches the light by the bed on. I recognise her. It's Kunju, the nurse who helped me the first night. "What is the matter, Gerald?"

"I have an awful pain." I tap my chest, I need something to take it away. Now. Please."

"I will see if I can get something for you."

"No! Don't see if you can get something—get me something! Now!" My voice is raised and there is irritation in it that I instantly regret.

"Don't raise your voice to me, Gerald, or be angry." She speaks quietly, "That will not help you. I am doing my best."

"Yes, I know you are, I'm sorry." I'm already feeling guilty, "I didn't mean to…I'm sorry, it's just that this pain is really hurting and… I want it to stop."

She moves away. "I will get something for you."

44

I lie back. The pain seems to be increasing and my guilt with it, my sharp words to her playing over and over in my head. I shouldn't have spoken to her like that. She *is* doing her best. The moaning starts again, it somehow lessons the discomfort, but I put my hand over my mouth to stop it and try to think of something, anything, to take my mind elsewhere… Heather… how good she is to me, what would I do without her… our trip to Madeira last year… … how she loved the ride on the Funchal cable car… the summerhouse we've built in the garden and how she helped us get the roof on… Cyril and me driving across America a few years ago… the fog enveloping the Golden Gate Bridge… the heatwave in New York… last Christmas with the family…

"Open your mouth, Gerald." Kunju is back. I open it and she squirts a liquid in. "That will help you," she says.

"What is it?" I ask.

"Morphine," she answers.

It does help, the pain lessens, and I fall asleep.

THURSDAY 30TH AUGUST

Cyril and Heather visited this afternoon and after they left, I endured an experience I don't want to experience again, the result of which is I now have a 'nasal gastric tube' up my nose, down my throat, and into my stomach. The tube is draining all the nasty stuff that has, apparently, settled there unable to move further due to the surgery. It is now flowing out—no, not flowing, trickling—out of my stomach, along the tube and into a plastic bag at the side of the bed. I stare down at it, a brown coloured obnoxious looking liquid. That stuff has been gathering in my stomach since last week. No wonder I have been feeling so bad, feeling sick and retching all over the place.

Inserting this gastric tube was an ordeal I do not wish to go through again. Two nurses came to my bed, one a very motherly type, Mary, talked a lot, the other younger, quieter.

"We need to insert an NGA line, Gerald, it's going to make you feel better," said Mary.

"Oh? What's that?" I asked, and she explained.

She held a thin plastic tube in her hand. "If you do exactly what we tell you it will be in and done in a few seconds. Can we go ahead?" I nodded. The younger one, Monique her name, handed me a glass of water, "Now," she said. "As Mary feeds it in you drink, okay?"

"Down my throat? What if I'm sick?"

"You won't be." Mary said as she advanced towards me and started to push the tube up my nostril. I jumped and pushed her hand away. It was almost instinctive. Having something pushed up your nose is not natural; it's not right. I don't like this.

"You've got to let me do it, Gerald. We'll go again, all right?" Monique says. I hesitate. They are both staring at me, waiting. I nod. This time I'm ready. "Drink," orders Monique. I put the glass to my lips, swallow some water. The tube is pushed up my nose; now it's in my throat, I want to gag, I pull back, the water spills, the tube comes out.

"I know this isn't pleasant," Mary says, "but we've got to get it in there, it really is necessary, I promise you. Let's try again."

They are both patient; it's obvious they have done this a thousand times before. They say the right things, words designed to calm, reassure. The tube is sliding down my throat again. My throat doesn't like it, my body doesn't like it, I don't like it.

"Drink!" ordered Monique. "More," says Monique, I drink more water. I want to retch. This is how I imagine waterboarding to be. I drink. I want this to be over.

I want Heather to be here. I want to go home.

"Nearly there, Gerald… drink." Mary says. I drink. The feeling of drowning again.

"Okay. We're there. Well done." Mary looks down at me, full of smiles. Monique squeezes my hand. "Good, this will make you feel better.

CHAPTER EIGHT

Copthorne Ward (continued)

The ward nurses change shift at ten o'clock. The night shift, six or seven nurses are led in by Shivani, and they all stop and form a half circle at the foot of my bed. Shivani clutches a clipboard and looking at it tells the group why I'm here, my condition, etcetera. A lot of medical jargon is involved. I notice Kunju, who catches my eye and give me a smile before they move on to next door Matt's bed area—which, as usual, has the screen around it.

Supper is brought, but I still have no appetite. I manage a little jelly and some ice-cream.

Blood pressure... Temperature... Pills... and then a porter turns up with a wheelchair. One of the nurses, Joe? Jim? Can't remember—tells me I am to be taken down to have my chest x-rayed to make sure the cough I have is nothing serious. I'm disconnected from all the lines, helped into the wheelchair, and off we go down to the X-Ray Department.

Along corridors, down a lift, past members of the public, visitors who glance at me, curiosity in their eyes; no doubt envy are in mine, they are going home tonight, fit and well… I will be here, not so fit, not so well.

Now we go through doors, and here we are. I'm parked outside for a few minutes and then wheeled in. This is where I came for the scan a few weeks ago. I'm X-Rayed and afterwards, a different porter takes charge of me. He says, "Copthorne, isn't it, mate?" I tell him, yes and he lets me know Copthorne is the furthest ward from the X-Ray Department. I'm not sure if he passes this information on to me to expand my knowledge of the geography of the hospital or if it's a complaint.

Back in Copthorne, Area 4, I am helped back into bed A, hooked up to the drip stand the plastic bag slowly filling with the contents of my stomach is placed at the side of the bed and I am left to sleep.

THURSDAY 30TH AUGUST

More pain. Not so bad as last night but intense enough to wake me up. It 1.30 AM. It's dark, I manoeuvre myself onto my back and the steady bleep… bleep… bleep of the machine at my side changes to a high-pitched urgent—don't ignore me—beep! beep! beep! beep! beep!

I stare up at the ceiling wondering if I should use the call button, but I'm saved that decision as footsteps approach.

"What's the matter, Gerald? A nurse I haven't seen before. She switches the light on and Fiddles with the machine attached to the drip stand and the URGENT beep! beep! beep! returns to the steady bleep… bleep… bleep…

"Try to keep your arm still or it will set off again, okay?" She says.

"Can you give me something for the pain?" I say and tap my chest.

"When did you last have paracetamol? You can't have more now if it's less than four hours ago."

"It's more than that."

"I'll check. I'll come back." She leaves me. I stare up at the ceiling again trying to concentrate on something other than the hurting which is now a dull intense ache more than a sharp pain.

From behind the screen next to me, I hear a groan, then an oath, a rattle of a wheelchair; Matt appears, glides past, stops at the little wash basin by the doors, cleans his teeth vigorously, and then wheels himself out of the area and disappears. It's nearly two in the morning.

The nurse comes back, shoots some paracetamol into me. I point to the screened bed next to me, "Where's he gone?" I ask.

"Cigarette," she says. "Or something like it." The aching pain recedes. I fall asleep.

I'm getting used to the routine. Blood pressure taken every two hours…temperature… Isabel with early morning tea… night shift handing over to the day shift…breakfast (though I still have no appetite and can only manage a few spoonful's of porridge)…bed changing… wash…drug trolley… (drink that water, Gerald!)… doctors' visit, a different one today, Mr Tim Piggot-Smith, "How are you feeling?" He asked. "This is a setback for you, I know, but it will come right… Have you opened your bowels? No? Any wind? No? It'll happen, just give it time… "

I'm hardly aware of the NGA line down my throat which surprises me, but the flow through it seems slow and intermittent. The plastic bag at the side of the bed is barely a quarter full. I still feel lethargic and weak, and it is an effort to be social. I haven't spoken to any of the other three patients here, just nodded 'hello.' I still feel ill—not so ill as yesterday and the days before yesterday—but rough. One of the booklets they gave me before I came in here said, "Most people feel tearful on the fourth or fifth day after surgery." I don't feel like crying but I do feel depressed, or maybe I am just feeling sorry for myself. I've got to snap out of it.

Chris, in the corner, is going home today. "Okay to have a shower?" He asked Jo, the nurse in charge today. "'Course," she said, and he goes into the bathroom and fifteen minutes later comes out looking clean and fresh and ready for home and shouting, "Quick, nurse! The place is flooding!"

Water follows him out of the door, spreading across the floor. Jo is talking to James, and she looks up, "Oh my god!" She exclaims and dashes into the bathroom shouting, "Get a cleaner!" She emerges a few minutes later looking dishevelled but triumphant. "The drain was blocked," she announces. "Lucky my husband is a plumber and I know what to do."

At four o'clock, Heather walks in smiling as usual though I can see she is still concerned but positive as ever. She says, "You're looking better than you did yesterday, Tott. I think you are on the mend." I don't feel as if I'm on the mend. "I hope you are right," I say. "Where's Cyril?"

"We're going to take it in turns visiting if it's all right with you, me today, your brother tomorrow. Do you mind?"

"No, that's okay. Makes sense."

CHAPTER NINE

A leak from the join?

FRIDAY 31ST AUGUST 2015

I'm woken by gunfire. It's coming from the screened-off bed area next door. Someone is shouting. More gunfire, more shouting, "Give it up, Jo!"

My sleep-filled head clears. Matt has the television on. It's "Rawhide" or "The Ponderosa" or could be "Wagon Train". I think I heard Ward Bond's voice, but whatever it is why the hell is it on at this time of night? It must be two o'clock in the morning. Why doesn't he use earphones?

Thoughtless, selfish, self-centred sod.

It's still a negative answer each time I am asked, 'Have you opened your bowels, Gerald?' and I'm becoming concerned. In the 'Enhanced Recovery Programme' booklet given me, it says, 'Severe pain that lasts several hours may indicate a leak from the join in the bowel. This is an uncommon complication but can be very serious.' This only happens in 5% of cases. Could I be in that 5%?

Shift change-over. The nurse in charge last night, an older lady I haven't seen before, reels off my condition to her day shift colleagues, most of which I don't understand or can't hear. She ends with a number, apparently, I was 'One' last night. I'll have to ask what that means.

Isabel comes round with her breakfast trolley. I force myself to eat some porridge and jelly and drink some orange and a glass of water. I still have no appetite, and it takes me a long time to get it all down. I am still feeling weak and lethargic.

Chris, the chap that was in the corner has been discharged and a new man has replaced his position, Darren his name, in his forties, I would guess. The screens have been pulled around his bed and the Stomer nurse is spending time with him, so obviously, he's here for bowel problems that are more serious than mine. I am not feeling as bad as I did yesterday, but I'm still not right. The pain seems to come and go, and I feel so weak. Still, it is only eight days since the operation, and I was told there would be a three-month recovery period, so I suppose I am being an impatient patient.

The bed-changers came round earlier and helped me into the chair in the corner, drip stand by my side, then it was the drug trolley with well-spoken Mathew, "Good morning, Gerald. How are you feeling today? Have you any pain?" Pills in a small plastic cup. Paracetamol into my arm.

I've become a little confused with everything. there have so many things been happening to me, so I spent some time this morning staring up at the ceiling, trying to work things out. The plastic bag at the side of the bed with the tube that leads into my stomach is now half full of the horrible looking brown sludgy stuff. Better in there than in me, but it means my bowel isn't working. Did they explain this to me when they shoved this tube down my throat? Maybe they did, and I didn't take the information in. I think I was too concerned about what was about to happen to me at the time, but it doesn't matter, Mr Smith ('call me Neil') and his team came round earlier and he explained what was occurring—or not occurring is a better description.

"The bowel doesn't like to be touched," he informed me, "and sometimes, and it's happened with you, when it is touched it goes to sleep and it is a matter of time before it wakes up again. It may take a day or two; it's difficult to predict, but it will wake up and things will return to normal."

He smiled his everything-is-going-to-be-all-right-don't-worry-smile, and he and his team moved on to the new chap, Chris, in the corner.

Well, no leak from the join then. If there was any hint of that he would have mentioned it, wouldn't he? 'Course he would. He's the expert. He's doing this every week. Operating every week, three or four times; he knows bowel cancer inside out, back to front, from the large bowel to the rectum, from the small bowel to the anus. I have no need to worry.

The old boy opposite me, James (perhaps I should stop calling him 'the old boy' as I have just found out he is the same age as me) after the doctor's tour and it was all quiet, started to shout, "Nurse!

Nurse!" but there was no response and after a couple of minutes he shouted again. He sounded distressed so grabbing hold of the drip stand, we manoeuvre over to him, "What's up, James?"

"I've lost the bloody emergency button, and I want to go to the toilet," he said in a querulous tone. The button was on the floor hanging from the side of the bed I picked it up and handed it to him. "There you go," I said wondering whether I should offer to help him into the toilet, quickly deciding against that idea. Over the last three or four days I had observed, too many times, nurses helping him into the toilet, holding, for modesty reasons, the hospital gown he wore across his pale, scrawny backside. No, I'm not doing that, I decide, and drip stand, and I move back to my bed area with a slight feeling of guilt which evaporates when Shivani comes in and takes charge of him, all smiles. "Hello, James, are you all right? What do you want?"

Cyril came to visit in the afternoon. I wasn't feeling so good again, and although I tried, I wasn't too social. My brother tried to make conversation, but I found it hard to respond until he told me our half-brothers, Richard and his wife Gabby and Derek and his wife Pam are coming down over the weekend and would like to come and see me. I responded then but not positively. I should have. (They are travelling hundreds of miles and have asked to see me. How kind, how thoughtful!) But I didn't. I didn't want them to see me like this—attached to a drip stand, an NGA line up my nose leading into a bag of sludge; urine bottle on standby at the side of the bed… Can you put them off? I said. "Can you tell them I'm not up to it?" He agreed. "Okay," he said, "I'll talk to them, I'm sure they will understand."

After Cyril leaves, and feeling a little better, I decide to take a walk, so drip stand by my side, we move slowly out of Area 4 and into the main thoroughfare of Copthorne Ward; bed areas off to my right and left, I glance into each. One looks like all women, another, old men. I keep walking, rather slowly past the reception counter. The two nurses there glance up at me, smile, one says, "Going for a walk? That's good. Don't get lost!"

I make my way out to the main corridor and sit on one of the seats, thoughtfully placed, I guess, for people like me who must sit down and rest after a couple of hundred steps. I gaze out of the window. The weather looks good, little white clouds, patches of blue. I sit and watch the passing parade: two doctors deep in conversation walk by, a cleaner with brooms and mops and other paraphernalia attached to his cart, wheels slowly past, two junior female nurses come out of the nearby lift, one leaning close to the other and speaking quietly into her colleague's ear. As they drew level I heard, "What do you think, should I? Would you?" The words creating all sorts of possibilities in my mind and visions in my head.

Two visitors come past, middle-aged ladies, one carrying a sad-looking Tesco bag the other is more up-market, she has an M&S bag in her hand with smart looking rope handles. "She looks much better now, don't you think?" Says one.

"Oh, yes, they've worked wonders, did you see her last week?" Says the other. "She was at death's door, I swear it."

None of these people glance my way. They probably don't even notice us, me, and drip stand, sitting here, me in my PJ bottoms, tee shirt, slippers, and pullover. We make our way back to Copthorne

Ward, Area 4, bed A and arrive in time for supper—and I force some jelly and ice cream down and a cup of tea. Then it's drugs time, then blood pressure measurement time again, not forgetting, 'Have you opened your bowels today, Gerald?'

CHAPTER TEN

An NGA line

SATURDAY 1ST SEPTEMBER

I wake, and the pain is back. I peer down at the plastic bag by the side of the bed that the NGA line is supposed to be feeding, I can hardly see it in the gloom, but it doesn't look as if there is any more of the brown sludgy stuff in there than there was yesterday. That means stuff is in my stomach that shouldn't be there. Is that why it's hurting? I move my hand to my chest and the steady bleep...bleep... bleep of the machine feeding me nutrients changes to the urgent, loud, beep! beep! beep! I look up at the small screen, "Infusion stopped", it says, "check fluid path between pump and patient access site."

I feel around for the call button, find it, press it. Wait... At last, footsteps... The light by the bed is switched on, a figure fiddles with the machine, the urgent beeping stops and returns to the steady bleep... bleep... bleep...

"Hello, Gerald. What's the matter?" It's Kunju.

"I've got a pain," I touch my lower chest, "and this bag, it's not filling."

She picks the bag up and shakes it. "Mmm." She puts it down again but in a different position and twiddles around with the plastic line. "Okay, it's coming out now." I look down and can see gunge flowing along the tube and dripping into the bag.

"How bad is the pain?" She asks.

"It's not so bad now, I think it's easing," I say, and I think it is.

Darren, the new chap in the corner has been told he needs an NGA line inserted. I know this because as this is a small area with just four of us in it is easy to hear conversations going on around other beds and Darren has not been quiet in his resistance. "I'm not having it," he says, loudly. "Forget it. Down my throat? No way, it's out of the question!"

The nurses—several—have been trying to persuade him for most of the day but have so far failed. His wife has been here, back and forth. In her thirties, slim, dark hair, attractive. He is clearly in pain but seems determined. ("It's no good you keep asking me—the answer's no!")

At one stage, she came out from behind her husband's screened off bed, tears in her eyes, "I'm going, Darren. I can't stand this." And she clipped clopped out of our area in her high-heels, and I thought she had left and gone home, but a few minutes later, she came back but stood at the door to our enclave not far from where I was sitting up in bed reading (and feeling much better now, thank you.)

She stood there for a few minutes and caught my eye a couple of times and after a minute or two she came over, "May I ask you a question?"

"Yes, of course," I said. "That..." She hesitated and pointed toward my nose... "That tube thing you have... does it hurt... I mean when they put it in, is it difficult?"

"It doesn't hurt, no, but it isn't the most pleasant experience when it's inserted, but I'm glad it's there. I mean, if it wasn't all the stuff collecting in my stomach would be causing major problems. Tell your husband it is about twenty to thirty seconds of discomfort and then it's over. Once it's in, he will start to feel better."

"Thank you. I hope you didn't mind me coming over and asking—"

"No, I don't mind at all."

An hour or so later, the nurses had another go at persuading him and this time was successful. I could hear the procedure taking place. ("Drink, Darren, drink!) I tell myself my short chat with his wife had influenced him, but I don't really know if it did.

SUNDAY 2ND SEPTEMBER

Rowdy Yates wakes me. *"Okay, Mr Favor, I'll head out."* 'Rawhide,' Clint Eastwood pretending to be an 1860s cattle drive scout. Cow's mooing, horses galloping, music. It's the TV again; at two o'clock in the morning. Behind his screened off bed area Matt has the volume up too high and I also get a whiff of something, a cigarette? Something else? Surely not.

I start to turn over, beep! beep! beep! I look up at the machine I'm attached to, "Infusion stopped, check fluid path between pump and patient access site." Bloody thing.

Well-spoken Mathew comes along, switches the bed light on, presses buttons, the steady bleep... bleep... bleep... returns.

"It is very sensitive, Gerald. You should try to keep your arm still." Easier said…

I decide I'm going to complain about Matt's TV but then realise it's not on now, so I don't say anything.

"How are you feeling, Gerald? Any pain?" Mathew asks. I shake my head. No there is no pain. A metallic sound comes from behind Matt's screen, an expletive, followed by Matt in his wheelchair. He stops at the wash basin by the door, cleans his teeth vigorously and then rolls through the door and out of sight.

"Why does he keep the screen around his bed all the time?" I ask Mathew. Mathew shrugs his shoulders. "I don't know, he shouldn't really, but, well, he is a bit of a loose cannon."

Things are looking up. The cough seems to have gone. To the daily question, "Have you opened your bowels today, Gerald?' This morning I answered, "Yes, well, sort of. I mean there has been a southern wind, and a little diarrhoea."

The nurse, Annette, looked delighted. "That's good." She laughed, "Things are beginning to move. Make sure you tell us each time, we need to take samples."

In the middle of the morning Mr Piggott-Smith and a young man I hadn't seen before, a junior doctor I surmised, stopped by the bed with the usual questions: "How are you feeling now? Any nausea? Any wind? Have you opened…?" I answered positively: Much better, no, yes, yes.

He looked pleased picked up the bag at the side of the bed, studied the contents. "Mmm…" he murmured, "I think we will leave things as they are for a couple more days, okay?"

"Yes, fine, if that's what you think is best."

"Good," he said and nodded to his junior colleague who was shuffling some papers and looking puzzled. "Isn't this Mr Thompson?"

"No, this is Mr Thornhill. I suggest you make sure you are talking to the patient you should be talking to when you visit. Otherwise, it could become confusing for all concerned, wouldn't you agree, Mr Thornhill?"

I laugh. "I would agree, yes." The junior doctor looked a little sheepish as they moved over to Darren in the corner.

I feel much better, and the day has been going by quite merrily; I went for another walk, a little further this time, and I was much steadier on my feet. When I got back, I decided to have a good and thorough wash in the bathroom. I am unable to shower yet due to the cannulas in my arm and my drip stand friend, who follows me everywhere, so a good wash is the best I can manage, my hair looks lank, though I can't do much about that yet. But today's effort ended not quite so merrily. I had hooked my other constant companion, the plastic bag receiving the contents of my stomach, onto the drip stand and was trying to get it into a position that would enable me to wash reasonably thoroughly when the line caught itself on something, pulled out and fell to the floor. The Elastoplast stuck to my nose and holding the line in position had worked loose. I looked down at it with dismay—I knew I would have to go through the insertion procedure again, and sure enough, as I came out of the bathroom Shivani was there and said, "Where is the NGA line?"

I had it in my hand and held it up. "It came out while I was trying to wash."

"We will have to put it back in." I shrugged my shoulders and said okay, and sooner the better and a half hour or so later it was: "Drink, Gerald, drink!" And the same sensation of being water boarded for thirty seconds was with me again and then, once more, a tube was up my nose, and in my stomach and the nurses were smiling and saying, 'Well done, Gerald!' And I, for a reason I cannot fathom, was feeling immensely pleased.

Heather came in the early evening. I had fallen asleep in the chair, and I woke up and there she was, smiling down at me. "You are looking a lot better, Tott, you've got your colour back. How are you feeling?"

"Yes, much better," I say. Her being here with her smile makes me feel *very* much better. I should have told her that. Why didn't I?

CHAPTER ELEVEN

A tragic story

MONDAY 3RD SEPTEMBER

It looks as if next-door-behind-behind-his-screen-Matt is leaving us. I listened (couldn't help listening) to a conversation between him and Darren this morning.

Clearly, Darren is feeling much better now, he was out of bed and sitting by the window and Matt had wheeled over.

I picked up on the conversation as Matt was saying, "Yeah, well, I should-a gone 'ome a couple weeks ago, like, "but the bloody Social Services fucked that up for me."

"What happened?" Asked Darren.

They reckon they 'ave to come. I've got a boy—he's ten—so they're checking he's all right, it's just an excuse to stick their noses in. I've told 'em to fuck off before now. Anyway, I bought my boy a toy gun, you know, like a pistol, plastic, it's a toy. One of these stupid social service cows reports it to her supervisor, only she says it's a real gun, so they refuse to come until I get rid of it.

I told them not to be so bloody stupid—it's just a fucking toy, but then the police got involved and they came round and after a load of ridiculous arguments, agreed it was a toy, but still the social services wouldn't come so the hospital wouldn't release me until it was sorted."

"Have they sorted it now?"

"Yeah, they're going to, like, discharge me tomorrow.

A short silence and then Darren's voice, "What's put you in the wheelchair?"

"Huh, well, I'll tell yer. I was nineteen, me and me mate, we'd been out, picked a couple of girls up, 'ad a few drinks, like. We was coming home, me mate was driving, he'd had too many—well, we all 'ad 'ad too many. Comes to this roundabout, we're going too fast for it, and he oversteers the bloody thing; we hit the fuck'n roundabout, shoots across it, comes off the other side and hits a fucking lorry. Been in a wheelchair ever since."

"Christ! What happened to your mate and the two girls?"

"He was no mate of mine after that. Tried to blame me, tried to make out in court it was me driving, but the police prosecuted him—driving under the influence, dangerous driving, they threw everything at him. He got five years."

"Were the girls hurt?"

"Killed, mate." There was a silence. Darren probably as shocked as I was.

Matt again: "Anyway, I'm going for a fag, mate, See yer later." He wheels past me nods 'hello' and disappears out of the door.

They've taken one of the cannula's out, the one that was used to shoot paracetamol into me, so now I've just got one line attached to the drip stand and I've learnt how I can disconnect that, so this afternoon I went for another walk but this time without the companionship of drip stand. I even climbed up and down a flight of stairs, so things are looking up.

I've had several visitors today. Neil Smith and his team, "You are looking better, Mr Thornhill, how are you feeling?" Have you had any bowel movement?"

"Yes, I am. Yes, I have." Everyone looked pleased. He points to the line in my nose. "Perhaps we can take that out, Mr Thornhill." It's almost a question.

"I don't want you to do that if there is any possibility of it having to go back in—I don't want to go through that procedure again."

"All right, we'll leave it another day, okay?"

The pain nurse came along, introduced himself. Middle-aged, smiley. I could have done with you a few days ago, I thought. Didn't say. A man from the hospital radio came, "Have you any music requests?" Not today. Then a doctor, female, flawless brown skin, very white teeth, looked no older than eighteen but must have been in her mid-late twenties (she's a doctor, after all). She was slim, attractive, professional, friendly. She introduced herself, but I can't now recall her name. "I'm Doctor … " And she sat down and kind-of interviewed me. How was I now? On a scale of one to ten where would I put the pain I have had? When I go home is there someone to look after me? A dozen other questions I am unable to remember. Nor can I remember what department she was from. Part of Neil Smith's team I assumed, though I hadn't seen her before. (I would have remembered her; she was very attractive) she gave me an injection in my stomach. "To prevent blood clots," she said.

THURSDAY 6TH SEPTEMBER

Early morning, Matt has gone home, replaced by a Scot with a very strong accent. He is ex-army, he has "been all over." He told me, "Gibralter, Singapore, oh aye, dozens of places."

Shivani is taking my blood pressure, temperature, etc. I ask her, "When the night shift hands over to the day shift the nurse who's handing over always gives a figure when she or he finishes describing my condition, like, 'Gerald is one, or Gerald is one-and-a-half. What does that indicate?"

"You shouldn't talk while I'm taking your blood pressure, haven't I told you that before, Gerald?"

"Aren't you going to tell me, Shivani?"

"It's just a measurement of how your night went. Two not so good, one better."

She removes the blood pressure cuffs. "How is it?" I ask.

"It's okay."

"Are you sure? I mean, you being so close to me I thought it might be up a bit."

She looks at me and smiles, "If you are trying to flirt with me it isn't going to work."

"Are you married, Shivani?"

"Yes, and so are you."

"Oh—is that a reprimand?"

"Yes." I laugh as she packs her equipment up and wheels her cart away.

I had another shower this morning and washed my hair again. Things are getting back to normal. ('Have you opened your bowels, Gerald?' 'Yes.')

I went for another walk, ascended, and descended a flight of stairs. Back in the enclave I walk over to Darren and sit and chat. He is a taxi driver; he tells me and has had bowel problems for years. After his recent surgery, he now has a stoma, and the stoma nurse has been teaching him how to use it. "She's been terrific," he says. He was philosophical about the stoma. He shrugged his shoulders, "I'm getting used to it. It's better than the alternative." He hesitates for a second or two and then, "Have you...?"

"No," I say, and think how lucky I have been. Lucky Heather insists on me having check-ups and blood tests regularly; lucky this was diagnosed so early; lucky I live in the UK and we have the NHS...

I rang my sister, Stephanie. "How are you?" I ask.

"I'm okay, what's more important is how are you?"

"Good," I say. "Great," I say. "I'm feeling fine," I say.

FRIDAY 7TH SEPTEMBER 2018

Last day at East Surrey Hospital.

I have a shower, eat breakfast, sit and read as they change the bed, am given pills from the drug cart, chat to Darren, chat with James—he still doesn't know if there is a place for him in the home in Crawley—I speak to Ben, the new guy in the bed next door. "How are you doing?" I ask.

"I'm okay," he says in his thick Scottish accent. "Did I tell you I was in the army? Oh aye, twenty-five years, I went all over, Singapore, Gibraltar— "

"Yeah, you mentioned it," I say.

Shivani says to me, "You are going home today, Gerald."

"Yes," I answer and grin. "Will you miss me?"

She smiles, "Not a bit!"

While I was waiting for Heather and Cyril to pick me up, I got my laptop out and looked up a couple of statistics:

There are around 16,000 bowel cancer deaths in the UK every year (44 every day). It is the 2nd most common cause of cancer death in this country.

The most common is lung cancer.

I think back to the 30th of April and my attending the surgery in Lingfield. Dr Richardson staring at the computer screen and looking up at me, "You are a little anaemic, Mr Thornhill, we must find out why."

Well, we found out why and it was over now, feeling good, I was fine, back to normal.

Or so I thought…

CHAPTER TWELVE

A routine check-up

WEDNESDAY 13TH MARCH 2019

It was the 13th of March, at least it wasn't a Friday, not that I am superstitious. But it was the date this whole thing started up again. I went to East Surrey Hospital for a CT scan arranged by Neil Smith prior to seeing him for a routine check-up after the bowel surgery that I'd had the previous August. The surgery was successful. "I don't think there is a real need but with your permission I will keep an eye on you—a check-up every six months, is that okay?" Neil had said when I had last seen him a couple of weeks after being discharged.

So I had the CT scan, it was a Wednesday, I think. Never liked Wednesdays, never liked February, but anyway, it was another ride to East Surrey for another CT scan: "Breath in… Hold your breath… Keep still… Breath out…"

Now it's a few days later and with Heather, I'm sitting in the hospital waiting to see Neil Smith. I have no concerns. I'm not worried about anything; all is fine. They told me it would take three months to get over the bowel surgery which it probably did, but now I'm back to normal. I've been walking, cycling, enjoying. We are due to join Cyril at our place in Florida soon. Six weeks in the sun, relaxing, taking it easy, life is good, everything is good. Just a bit of a cough.

"Good to see you again. Sit down, make yourself comfortable." Mr Smith, his usual genial self, with a smile welcomes us. He introduces us to a girl sitting nearby, young teenager on work experience. "Okay," he says, "how are you?"

"Fine," I answer, "no problems, just a bit of a cough which seems to be hanging around, but apart from that…"

"I wanted him to go and see his doctor about that, but…" Heather said.

Neil fiddles with the computer, moves the mouse, peers at the screen. "Mmm…" He stood, "if we just go in here for a minute or two." He ushered me into a small side room where he examined my chest. Then it was back in front of his computer, and he swung it round so we could see the screen. He pointed at it and said, "That's the CT scan you had, that's your right lung, see that white spot there, at the top?" I nodded. "That showed up when you had the CT scan last year, remember?"

I nodded, yes, I remembered I had a chest X-ray just after the surgery because I had developed a cough which had kept me awake at night and they had sent me for an X-ray to "have a look."

"It doesn't seem to have got any bigger," Neil said, "but I think I'll put you on a course of penicillin which may clear it and to be on the safe side I'll arrange for you to have a check-up with the respiratory people. Okay?"

THURSDAY 16TH MAY

About three weeks later, Heather and I are sitting on hard plastic chairs in a waiting room of East Surrey Hospital. There were eight or nine of us sitting, there, all of us looking bored. A notice next to the reception desk told us, "Dr Nimako is running 30 minutes late." I looked for the letter that had come from the hospital but couldn't find it. "Is that who we are seeing?" I asked Heather. She nodded.

I'll never get used to this—sitting in hospital waiting rooms, waiting to be examined, X-rayed, poked at, questioned, scanned, and various other personal invasions. If it wasn't for Heather, always encouraging and supporting me, I'm not confident I would go through with all this. Up to last year's bowel cancer, apart from visiting friends and relatives I hadn't set foot in a hospital for seventy years. Now it seems to have become a regular occurrence. But I am now in my eighties so—and I write this reluctantly—I should expect it, but I didn't expect it, I think I thought I would carry on as normal, feeling fine, active, enjoying retirement, spending months of the year in sunny and warm Florida, and that's the way it would stay until I was in my nineties, and then...? Well, slip away as the Royals do, peacefully, in my sleep.

My name is called. A young lady, attractive in her twenties asked me to follow her, so Heather and I stand, and we are led into a small office-like room with three chairs grouped near to a computer. The young lady introduces herself and I instantly forget her name. She asks if I have ever smoked, and I tell he 'yes' but gave it up over forty years ago. She shrugs and in a gesture of dismissal smiles and says, "that's all right then." She makes small talk for a while and then Dr Nimako comes in, greets us, and sits by the computer and pulls up the latest CT scan I had, studies it for a while and then points to the white area at the top of my right lung.

"I think the best thing we can do now is for you to have a biopsy to see exactly if this is something nasty… or not." You would have to come in for a day, maybe overnight, though that isn't likely." He said.

"A biopsy?"

"Yes, we take sample, and it will tell us exactly what this is."

He picks the mouse up and slides it around the screen and after a couple of seconds, "We could have you in on the 22nd."

"The 22nd? I looked at Heather, "We are going out to our place in Florida next Friday, the 15th. We'll be away for six weeks."

There is a silence. Dr Nimako says, "Well, it's up to you."

He picks the mouse up again. Moves it around. What date will you be back?"

"We're back on the May 2nd, Doctor, Heather says.

He looked up from the screen, "We could see you on the 3rd of May, but I suggest you go away and think about it, if you decide to have the biopsy on the 22nd call us."

"Will six weeks make a difference?" I asked.

"Well," he hesitated. "It doesn't seem to have grown since August, so perhaps not."

"Okay, I'll go for the 3rd of May, the day after we get back. But if I change my mind between now and next week I'll ring."

We all stand and shake hands.

"I hope we've done the right thing," I say to Heather as we drive home.

"'Course we have. Some time in the sun will do you good—do us both good."

CHAPTER THIRTEEN

Biopsy

FRIDAY 3ʳᵈ MAY 2019

We're back from Florida, and I am sitting with Heather again in the waiting room in the X-ray department of the East Surrey Hospital and read the paperwork that accompanied the appointment instructions. "Do not eat anything from midnight… drink plenty of water… Please arrange for someone to collect you following your discharge…" A nurse appeared, smiling, foreign accent, east European I guessed, mid-thirties.

"Mr Thornhill? I will weigh you, okay?"

"Yes, okay."

We walked to a small cubicle, and she said, "What is your date of birth, Mr Thornhill?" I told her and stood on the scales; she measured my height and took my blood pressure. I returned to the waiting room. It wasn't crowded, no more than a dozen of us sat there. There was a constant flow of people walking through the area: nurses hurrying to somewhere else, patients wandering through and looking lost, doctors on important missions, porters come past pushing wheelchairs with elderly people slumped untidily in them.

"I've put on weight." I tell Heather, "six pounds. I'm not too happy about that."

"It's better than losing it in your condition, isn't it?"

I never thought of that.

The actual biopsy took about a half-hour. Dr Nimako warned me before he started the procedure that he might accidently touch one of my ribs and that might cause some discomfort.

He did touch them a couple of times, and it made me jump and it did cause some discomfort. It hurt like hell. Apart from that, the procedure wasn't too bad. After several minutes, he said," I've taken a few samples. I think that's enough."

THURSDAY 16TH MAY 2019

We get the result of the biopsy today. East Surrey Hospital again. Dr Nimako sat by his computer moving a mouse about. Heather and Cyril are with me. We all shook hands. There is a short silence. Then, "Well, Mr Thornhill, we have the result of the biopsy, and I'm afraid it's not good news. You have lung cancer, but it's operable. Before we get to that, I think you should have a lung function test and a Pet-scan and we'll include a brain scan to make sure nothing has spread, all right? After that, you won't see me again, but I'll arrange for you to see the surgeon, Mr Hunt, and that will be at St George's Hospital in London and he will arrange everything for you."

I am shocked and stunned. My thoughts are in a whirl. I feel much worse than when I was told I had colon cancer. This seems more final. "He's got lung cancer". In the past when I have been told that I have always thought it was just another way of saying he hasn't got long to go…

Haven't I got long to go? Dr Nimako asks if we have any questions. The thought crosses my mind to ask, 'How long have I got ?" But then I realize it could be insulting. He's just told me 'It's operable.' Meaning presumably, he can cure it, and anyhow I doubt he would tell me even if he has got an inkling. I can't think of any other questions, though I know when we get home I'll think of a dozen.

Heather asks, "When will he undergo the surgery?"

"You will be written to in about a week," was the answer.

Heather was her usual upbeat positive self on the way home. "They can operate, that's the main thing, Tott—and they are making sure it hasn't spread to other places and at least we will know you've got a brain."

I was trying to absorb the news, but it was difficult. Lung cancer—it sounds so final. How long have I got? That was what I wanted to ask but didn't. Maybe I was frightened of the answer. A short tussle goes on in my head. Should I ask or not? Do I really want to be told? What if the answer is six months? What would I do? Buy a few dozen packets of paracetamol, end it all? No, while there's life, there's hope – and that wouldn't be fair to Heather, anyway. So I push that thought aside.

A week or so later, I am invited to the Royal County Surry Hospital in Guildford for a 'Pet Scan on May 29th. My computer tells me "The PET scan uses a mildly radioactive drug to show up areas of your body where cells are more active than normal. It's used to help diagnose some conditions, including cancer. It can also help to find where and whether cancer has spread." This will be my second PET SCAN. I had one prior to my bowel op last year. It is all organised, handled and carried out by Alliance Medical who provide PET and CT scanning services across 30 locations in England. It crosses my mind that they may be part of the creeping privatisation of the NHS which the present government deny is occurring. I hope I am wrong.

THURSDAY 31ST MAY 2019

East Surrey Hospital (again!) today for a lung function test. This consists of breathing and blowing into a tube which presumably measures the efficiency of the lung, or perhaps in my case the inefficiency. It was conducted by a friendly man with the strangest of accents. "Where are you from?" I asked.

"Guess." He grinned.

"Somewhere in eastern Europe?"

He smiled. Shook his head. "Tasmania."

I have had several scans over the last few weeks, seen Mr Hunt, and me, Cyril, and Heather recently had a pleasant weekend in Felixstowe meeting up with half-brothers Richard and Derek and their wives. My sister, Stephanie, also joined us.

I've been given a date for admission to St Georges Hospital in London for my lung cancer operation. September 30th. How I wish today was 1st August and this cancer business was all over and finished with and life was back to normal.

MONDAY 1ST JULY 2019

Cyril driving, we travel up to, St George's Hospital in Tooting, London. It took about an hour. I looked it up. St George's is a teaching hospital, so I trust all those involved in my surgery have been well taught.

We make our way to the Caroline Ward on the third floor and are asked to wait in the waiting room which overlooks the car park we have just left. After a while I am asked into an annexe where a lady introduced herself as the anaesthesiologist who will be attending me during the surgery, which, she told me, is scheduled for tomorrow. She asked a lot of questions; none I can remember now, and then told me they are getting my bed ready, and I will be moved into the ward shortly. I return to the waiting room and tell C and H they may as well go home as nothing else will be happening today, but they stay until I am settled into the ward. I lounge on the bed, which is by the window, next to me a chap fast asleep. Opposite an elderly guy who is being visited by—I guess—his daughter.

Mr Hunt, my surgeon, visited and asked how I was feeling and told me I was on his schedule for tomorrow afternoon. My blood pressure was taken; I sent a text to H and C to tell them I was settled in and had been given a meal. Through the window it was twilight and feeling a little bored, I decide to go for a walk. I passed a shop on the ground floor, but it had no interest to me, and I strolled through the car park and out to the road. It's not a particularly attractive area, but I walked for a few minutes around the block and back into the hospital passing on the way a pub with its doors open and the sound of conversation, clinking of glasses, and laughter emanating from the interior. For a few seconds I was tempted to go inside and have a pint as the thought struck me it could be my last opportunity—and it could be my last pint! But then decided as I was having a major operation tomorrow it was not a good idea.

I returned to the ward.

CHAPTER FOURTEEN

Lobectomy

TUESDAY 2nd JULY 2019

I slept well, and this surprised me a little. I'm having a lobectomy today, so I should be worried, shouldn't I? That thought sets me thinking more deeply which wasn't good because they drift to what-if-something-goes-wrong thoughts and today, July 2nd 2019 is the date some stonemason somewhere will be taking a note of before he starts carving it into a piece of what? Marble perhaps? I quite fancy black marble, gold letters:

Gerald Hugh Thornhill

7th April 1937 – 2nd July 2022

An honest and decent man.

Have I been honest and decent? I like to think so. Not always honest maybe, but mostly decent. I can call myself that. With honesty. Another thought has just floated in. What if the surgery this afternoon doesn't clear all the cancer and I must go through months of taking pills, having radiation and chemotherapy and god know what else. The chemo is the most concerning. I have read a patient can expect to have side effects of nausea, vomiting, neurotherapy, constipation, have trouble breathing, a weakened immune system, possible hair loss, depression, aggression, anxiety, and probably other effects not talked about.

Chemotherapy was mentioned to me last year in connection with the bowel cancer, though I was assured the decision to have it, if it was thought necessary, would be mine. It wasn't necessary then, and I hope it won't be this time. But if I was told you have it or you only have six months to live, I suppose I might see things in a different light. What if they said a year?

No.

Two years?

No.

So how long is acceptable? It's one of those questions I don't want to examine, so I'm not going to, and I won't answer it. I don't want to think about chemotherapy, radiotherapy, and other means of messing about with my body to make it better again.

These last few years of retirement have been fantastically good, and I trust this time tomorrow I will be able to look forward to happy times once more.

In the afternoon somewhere around three o'clock, I am wheeled up to a small room which I assume is next to the operating theatre. I'm nervous. A woman comes in, her head wrapped in what could be a hijab, though it may be just a headscarf. If it's a hijab, does it mean she is a Muslim. What difference does that make to me, anyway?

None. She smiles down at me, and I realize she is the anaesthetist who spoke to me yesterday. She stands at the head of the trolley, "How are you feeling?" She asks. I tell her I'm feeling fine, and she smiles again. Now it's a repeat of last August, my heart rate, blood pressure, and oxygen level are taken; a young chap who doesn't look old enough to do what he is doing inserts a cannula in my arm, the anaesthetist makes small talk, I can't recall a word she said to me, then, just like last August, I start to feel dizzy, and then a little distant, sound becomes muffled and then... darkness.

* * *

A nurse is taking my blood pressure. She asks me my date of birth; do I feel sick? Have I any pain? There are plastic tubes in my nose. Oxygen.

"Seventh of April, 1937" I say and "No, no."

About eight in the evening, Heather and Cyril are by the bed.

"How are you feeling?" They ask almost simultaneously.

"Yeah, fine." I said. And I did feel fine despite the fact Mr Hunt has removed one third of my right lung.

I'm not on oxygen now, and we walk together down to the garden area on the ground floor and sat on one of the benches for a while. I'm a little slow walking. But then, as I often say to myself, what's the hurry? When you examine things there isn't any really. There is little need to rush around the way we seem to do these days. Why do we do it? What *is* the hurry?

The weather was lovely while we sat there. Bright sunlight, blue sky, warm. There was a half-dozen or more patients and visitors also sitting enjoying the garden, chit-chatting. It was a pleasure to be there in the sunshine talking to Heather and Cyril. It was very agreeable for what could have been a last day on this earth.

WEDNESDAY 3RD JULY

Breakfast. I am in Godstone ward. Earlier, I heard a couple of nurses talking, and from what they said, it seems I might be moved. Caterham Dean was mentioned, which was where Heather spent some time after her hip operation. It's a little like a cottage hospital as they used to be so if that is where I do end up it will be fine with me.

The guy in the next bed is still asleep. A nurse has tried to wake him several times, but he's dead to the world. Not literally. He is breathing. They must have him on drugs.

In the middle of the morning, Mr Hunt and his team visit. He asks how am I feeling? Am I in any pain? Do I feel sick? No pain, I tell him, not sick, feeling fine. He and the team look pleased. It's true. I do feel fine. It doesn't seem as if I had a serious op just a few hours ago. He tells me it all went well, and he can't see why I shouldn't go home at the weekend.

I sort out my laptop and do some writing. Heather and Cyril visit. I tell them I could be coming home at the weekend. Heather pulls a face. "It's a bit soon, isn't it, Tott? Look what happened last time." (Last time, after the bowel cancer op, I was discharged within a couple of days of the surgery, and the next day was rushed back in by ambulance, very ill, and confined to the hospital for a further week.)

"We'll see what happens at the weekend," I say, "but right now I feel good."

"Yes, we'll see," Heather said. "But we don't want the same thing that happened last time to happen again, do we? You remember how ill you were, don't you? Are you sure you *are* okay?" I can tell she is not convinced as she still has a worried look on her face and is not smiling or as chatty as normally.

I do remember how ill I was, (see chapter 15 page 57 'Relapse') but I'm sure I want to go home, even though it was only yesterday I had the surgery. I reject the doubt that is creeping in.

This afternoon a doctor came to see me—I can't remember his name, though he must have told me—after talking for several minutes and answering his questions he decided I can be discharged today, and he is sorting out the paperwork. Heather and Cyril arrive. When I tell them what I thought was good news, Heather looks more worried. "Are you really sure, Tott? How do you really feel?"

I tell her. I feel good. Fine. No pain, no sickness, but I can tell she is not convinced. She still has a worried face and is not chatting. Always a sign she has stopped being the usual upbeat and happy Heather.

The release paperwork seems to take ages, but at last the ward sister comes up with it. Heather goes to the dispensary to collect the drugs I must take, home with me, and we are on our way. It's a beautiful day, sunny and warm. The journey seems to take twice as long as when we came on Monday, and the nearer, we get to East

Grinstead the more potholes we seem to hit. By the time we are home sitting and watching television together, I am not feeling quite so exuberant as when we left Tooting. Both H and C advise me to go to bed as I'm looking tired. I readily agreed.

CHAPTER FIFTEEN

Relapse

THURSDAY 4ᵀᴴ JULY 2019

A pain in my chest woke me. It's dark outside, must be around midnight. I pulled myself into a sitting position, and now I'm breathing hard but don't seem to be getting enough air into my lungs, and the pain is getting worse. I can feel the stirring of panic and feel for the bedside light switch. Did I bring my mobile up? Yes, thank heavens—there it is on the bedside table. I punch in Cyril's number.

"Hello, what's up?"

"I've got a bad pain, and I can't get my breath; I think I need an ambulance."

Heather came up. "Where is the pain?" She asked. I pointed to my chest. I didn't want to talk. The breathlessness seemed to be getting worse, and I was now getting into a panic. Cyril came into the room. "Ambulance on its way," he said.

"I need oxygen. I said. I'm breathing quickly. In-out-in-out-in-out. I'm conscious of them watching me. I don't know what to do. Heather hands me a glass of water and two pills. "Take these," she says. "They gave them to me at the hospital, they should stop the pain."

"How long will it be?" I say to Cyril.

He shrugged. "They said it's on its way."

"They might send a paramedic." Heather said. "It's quicker, one man in a car."

That's what they did. After about fifteen minutes, the doorbell rang and Reece, young, Australian accent, cheerful demeanour with large medical bag comes up to the bedroom. He asked a lot of questions. After a while, he said he wasn't too happy with my heart rate and if it were okay with us, he would get the 'waggon' and whisk me back to the hospital. No more than five minutes later, the ambulance arrives with two medics, one male, one female.

"Do we need the chair?" the girl asked.

"Can you manage the stairs?" Reece asked me.

I nodded. I was now breathing normally, but the pain persisted. I was loaded into the ambulance, and we set off. "We'll follow in the car!" Cyril shouted before the ambulance door slammed.

The journey takes a long time, but time has suddenly slowed to half its normal speed. Five minutes takes at the very least fifteen. A side effect of the pain, I think. The two medics check me every few minutes and make small talk, but I find it too difficult to respond— another side effect. We reach the hospital, and I'm shunted into an assessment ward. It's small, only a few beds, most of them empty. A nurse takes my temperature, heart rate, blood pressure, and hands me a plastic container with two pills in it and a glass of water. "Take these." She says.

After a few minutes, Heather and Cyril come in. Cyril finds a couple of chairs.

"How's the pain?" Heather asks.

"Bloody awful," I want to say, but don't. I just shake my head. It is now dominating my thoughts; I can't think of anything else apart from this persistent throbbing ache in my chest. I look around hoping to see a nurse or doctor rushing over to give me something to stop it. Another pill, an injection, anything for heaven's sake. A few minutes go by. "You should go home." I manage to say, "They'll look after me now."

Cyril shakes his head. Heather says, "No, we'll stay until we know what they are going to do. I've brought some things for you." She points to a bag on the floor. "Some PJs, toothpaste, shampoo, your laptop, kindle, phone and stuff." She grasps my hand, "Is it still bad, Tott?"

Yes, it bloody well is, I don't say. Just keep silent. Heather stands, looks round. "This is no good. I'll see if I can find someone."

Cyril and I sit in silence for a while. Then, "They sent you home too early."

I nod. He's dead right there. I should have taken note of Heather's doubts.

Heather comes back. "Someone is going to come and see you, Totty."

Time crawls. Nurses walk past. A woman pushing a trolley with crockery on it rattles by. The pain has eased a little.

Then, "Mr Thornhill?"

I nod as Heather says, "Yes."

A lady doctor is looking down at me. She introduces herself, and almost instantly, I forget her name. "We're trying to locate your paperwork. You are experiencing some pain, yes?"

"Yes"

"Where?"

I point to my chest.

"On a scale of one to ten, ten being the worst, where would you put it?"

"Eight to nine."

"He only had the surgery on Tuesday." Heather said.

"Tuesday?" She frowned. "Okay, the doctor who can administer a strong pain prevention, which I think you should have, is upstairs at the moment dealing with a critically ill patient. I'll get her here as soon as I can. Okay?"

I nodded. She left us.

Heather said, "Well, that's good. I'm sure they'll sort you out now, Tott."

"Course they will." Said Cyril.

I nod again. Tried to smile. Failed. Looked at my watch. It was five past one. "You should both go home." I said. "It's gone one. The pain has nearly gone."

"Are you sure? You don't mind?"

"No, 'course not. I'll see you tomorrow." Heather kisses me. They leave.

I looked around the immediate area. There were about five beds. Only three of them are occupied, each of the occupiers seem to be asleep; a distance away I can hear some sort of machine beeping, footsteps clip clop across a hard floor, the rattle of screens being pulled around a bed. Two nurses are laughing somewhere nearby, I assume they are nurses I can't actually see them.

The pain has lessened considerably, it is nowhere near as bad as it was when it woke me, which is now several hours ago. I doze.

* * *

"Mr Thornhill?"

I wake. A woman was looking down at me, round faced, smartly dressed. "Hello, I'm Doctor Hutchins. I'm going to take your blood pressure, is that okay?"

I nod. "Yes, fine."

She fiddles with the blood pressure cuff, wraps it around my upper arm, and I feel it tighten. A few seconds go by, and it relaxes and she writes something down.

"Is it okay?" I ask.

"Yes, I'm going to put the cannula in now."

On a one to ten scale, how is the pain now?"

"It's not so bad now, thank heavens, about six or seven."

She rubs some antibiotic on to my wrist. There is a small table by her side with an array of medications scattered across it. She pulled out one of the packaged needles, tore off the plastic wrapping, tapped my wrist looking for a vein. "This will pull a little." She said. I felt the prick of the needle. "Okay, that should ease things for you. We'll move you to a ward in a while. I'll just take your temperature. She pushed something against my ear and wrote something down, looked at me for a while as if trying to assess my character. And then said, "Try and get some sleep, Mr Thornhill."

CHAPTER SIXTEEN

A paravertebral nerve block

FRIDAY 5TH JULY 2019

It's several hours later. The scare of yesterday is over. I'm in a ward with about 20 beds with subdued lighting, something electric is humming, a machine is beeping, and someone is snoring. The pain has almost gone, and there is just an ache in my chest as if to remind me where it was and if it comes back that's where it will be. I wanted to pee and looked around hoping there was a toilet nearby. A few yards away, toward the end of the ward, there is a wide corridor with doors off to the right, and I guess one of them will lead into a bathroom. I pulled myself up and swung my legs out of the bed and stood letting a few seconds go by assessing the situation as I held on to the side of the bed. I felt okay. A little weak but confident I could walk and to prove it to myself took a couple of steps to the end of the bed. No problem.

I set off. Walked slowly, reached the wide corridor. Further along, a nurse is sitting at a lit desk writing. I stopped at the first door, and as I opened it, the nurse looked up. The door opened into a bathroom. I peed and walked back into the corridor. The nurse at the desk shouted, "Excuse me, what are you doing?"

She sounded autocratic. I walked towards her. "I needed the toilet," I said.

"You must not wander around like that, if you need help press your buzzer. Please return to your bed."

I had been reprimanded. I returned to my bed and slept for another hour or more. When I woke, the ward was coming to life. Breakfast was being served. I had some porridge, and as I was drinking a cup of tea, a male nurse came over. He shook my hand. "Hello Gerald, I'm nurse Trevor, how are you feeling?"

"Okay," I said.

"Have you been sick?"

"No."

"That's good. I'm in charge here if you need anything just call me."

"Does my wife know where I am?" I asked.

"Yes, she rang in."

The drug trolley came round, and I was given some pills to take. My temperature, oxygen, sugar level, and blood pressure were taken. It seems I am in the Critical Assessment Ward. Being assessed. Critically. Once that is accomplished, they will decide what to do.

There is someone the other side of the ward who keeps shouting, "Oh Lord!" Oh Lord!" I can't make up my mind whether he keeps being shocked or surprised by something he doesn't expect, or he's a religious nutcase (RN). I fear it is the latter.

Heather and Cyril visit. Heather is still looking worried. Cyril is not saying too much. The pain has come back, and I find it difficult to pretend all is well. I don't think I would ever win a medal for courage in adversity.

The nurse comes by to give me another injection. C and H make conversation. They tell me about the new restaurant they visited the other night, but I start to lose concentration and fall asleep. The next few hours are confused. I awoke in a small cubicle, no more than ten feet by six, blue curtains surround the bed. Two doctors were at the foot, one of them talking to me in a committed tone. He had an accent, German, I decided. His friend hardly spoke but when he did, he too sounded German.

Heather and Cyril are also here. Heather's hand is resting on my shoulder; she is smiling down at me, listening to the doctors, nodding in agreement to what they are saying. Cyril too is concentrating on what is being said. The quiet one of the two doctors leans closer to me and says, "Do you understand, Gerald? Should we go ahead?"

"No, I don't. What do you want to do?"

"It's called a paravertebral nerve block. It will take the pain away."

"It will? Really?"

"Yes, I promise it will."

Heather takes hold of my hand and squeezes it. "I think you should have it, Tott."

"Okay, if it's going to take this pain away, it's all right with me."

The doctor who had been talking to me picked up a clipboard and wrote something down. His colleague moved away through the blue curtain, and I heard a nearby door open and close. Then I noticed Cyril was standing to the left of the foot of the bed. He caught my eye, "Yes, you should have it, Gerald," He said. He is serious, I know because he doesn't often call me Gerald.

The two doctors push through the curtains, and I hear the door open and close again, then I heard Heather say to Cyril. "What do you think, Granddad?"

I didn't hear his answer.

Next, I am back in Godstone Ward. No pain. A nurse came over pushing a trolley, "How are you feeling, Gerald?"

I was feeling fine. "Good, thank you."

"I have to take your blood pressure, and there are some pills here for you." She picked up the water jug on the bedside table and poured some into a glass, handed it to me and with it a plastic holder containing three pills. She took hold of my arm and attached the cuff. I swallowed the pills. As she wrote down the blood pressure result, I asked if it was okay. She rattled off a set of figures that didn't mean a thing to me. "Is that good?" I asked and she said it was 'okay.'

Opposite my bed was a brick wall. The bricks were shiny, white, glazed. As I stared, they started to change colour, one by one, row by row, from white to blue to green to red, then they shivered and dissolved into a myriad of coruscating patterns, like a kaleidoscope. I was fascinated and couldn't move my eyes away. As I watched each began to disappear, one row at a time, slowly revealing the ward next door, which was busy. There were two doctors standing talking to one another, someone was shouting, the words incomprehensible.

The nurse loaded her equipment back onto the trolley, as she did, said, "Are you ready, Gerald?"

"Ready?" I said, puzzled. "What for?"

"We're all going out to dinner."

Out to dinner? This was a surprise to me. "Really?" I said. "Nobody told me. Could I have a couple of Paracetamol? The pain is creeping back. Should I change?"

"Don't worry, it will go away again in a minute or two. There's no need to change your clothes."

* * *

The minibus we were in was much like the 12-seater I used to drive for Don's Coaches in the sixties when I lived in Bishops Stortford. I was assigned it one Saturday and sent to Stansted to pick up a family and take them to Yardley Hastings in Northamptonshire for a wedding. The family included two uncles of the bride and a couple of female cousins. When we got there, Uncle Charlie, a jovial, friendly man insisted I join them at the reception and that was how I got to know his daughter, sixteen at the time, very pretty, long dark hair, beautiful smile…Heather.

CHAPTER SEVENTEEN

A night out

I sat, hunched up by the mini-bus window watching the passing scene. It was early evening, still light, weather fine. The roads were busy. Traffic lights and traffic jams, horns blaring, the pavements crowded with early evening shoppers, and workers scurrying home.

"Where are we?" I asked nobody.

"Redhill." A male voice answered.

At the restaurant we didn't sit together, we were scattered to various tables. Mine was up a step making me a little higher than everyone else and giving me a good view of the room. Over to the left of me were the two German doctors who had performed the paravertebral nerve block procedure on me earlier. They were at a table together and had a third man with them. They were both talking to him earnestly, and I gained the impression they were trying to persuade him to have the same process.

We were there for a couple of hours. I found it agreeable and fun. At one stage it became quite noisy. People shouting to one another, the nurses chatting to us. Raucous laughter, giggling. Every now and then one of the nurses would come over to me and ask, "Are you all right, Gerald?" I was all right. I was fine. The evening was a fantastic success as far as I was concerned. How good, I thought, that the hospital should go to the trouble of taking us out like this. It was certainly good for the morale.

But then the pain came back. Slowly and hardly noticeable at first just a little ache, not to be taken seriously. I tried to ignore it. But after a few minutes that became impossible. It was insidious. Artfully sending a one second piece of agony-stabbing pain every two or three minutes. It wasn't to be ignored. So much for the paravertebral nerve block procedure, I thought and looked across at the two German doctors hoping they would see me and come over to check how I was. I would then be able to tell them, and maybe they could stop these one second shots of pain which were turning the evening into misery. A wailing noise started. It was coming out of _my_ mouth. I quickly put my hand over it to suppress the noise I was making. People were looking, a nurse hurried over. "What's the matter, Gerald?"

"It's this bloody pain," I said, tapping my chest. "It keeps coming back. I'm sorry."

"You don't have to apologise. It will go away in a few seconds. Honestly, it will."

"How do you know?"

She smiled, a wide reassuring smile, "I'm a nurse, that's how. We're leaving in a minute or two, okay?"

SATURDAY 6TH JULY

I woke up back in Godstone Ward. It must have been in the early hours. Something had pulled me out of sleep. It wasn't pain; thank heavens, that seemed to have gone again. No, it was another patient, "Oh God, I pray to you! "Oh God, I pray to you!" He shouts.

Oh God, that's all I need. He keeps repeating it over and over, to the extent I imagine God is as fed up with hearing it as I am. After a while there are footsteps tap, tap, tapping across the floor. "Be quiet, Geoffrey. You are disturbing everyone!"

She can say that again.

Nurse Trevor came to see me. "How are you?" He asked. Yes. Okay, I told him. He took my blood pressure, temperature, etcetera, and made small talk to the background accompaniment of the ritual of "Oh God, I pray to you!"

I said, "Can't you shut that guy up? Shoot him or something?"

Nurse Trevor smile ruefully. "He's what you would call a cross we have to bear, I'm afraid."

Heather and Cyril visited this afternoon. While we are chatting, flies are around the bed. Large, black, ugly things. I keep swotting them away. Heather looks at me strangely. "Are you all right, Tott?" she asked.

"Flies." I mutter. "Shouldn't be here."

We went for a walk again. I feel okay, reasonably strong. We walk out of the ward, down the stairs past the shop and into the garden area. The sun is out again and there are several people sitting there, drinking tea, chatting. We sit together. I look around and realize, as I didn't last week, that this is the garden area in East

Surrey Hospital. I'm not back at St George's Hospital in Tooting where I believed the ambulance brought me the other day. No, I'm back in East Surrey, it's a bit of a shock and takes some getting used to. I didn't say anything to Heather and Cyril. I waited until they had gone and then spend some time thinking about it. I wonder if I've got a mental problem. Things are happening around me I don't understand. Time is floating past and yet everything seems a little distant, out of focus. I don't think I have felt like this before, and now for no reason I can fathom an incident from years ago goes through my head, like a film trailer.

One freezing winter morning, riding to work on my scooter, I hit a patch of ice and lost balance. The scooter clattered down the road in one direction. I slid in the other. It replays in my head like a film trailer. The clattering sound is muted, but the picture is high definition. It's a little like this hospital experience. Last year when I was in East Surrey for colon cancer, everything was crystal clear to me. I knew what was happening all the time. I could remember everything, every incident. This time, it's all muffled, subdued, distant.

A nurse interviewed me this evening. Another one whose name entered my brain for two or three seconds and quickly found an exit. She was a welfare person and asked a lot of questions about my circumstances. What sort of house I lived in, who with, how many stairs, did we have a garden? Any second I expected her to ask if I kept a mistress but that didn't seem to occur to her. After a fifteen-minute interrogation, she seemed satisfied I will be looked after when I return home and left me saying she will be back to see me again when I will need to practice going up and down stairs. That's okay, I know I can manage that.

Heather didn't look so worried on her visit with Cyril this afternoon. But that changed when I told by them about the evening out on Friday. They both listened to my description—the coach ride, the restaurant, seeing the two German doctors again, the nurses. When I finished, Heather was frowning and looking worried again. I said, "What's the matter, Bumble?"

She said, "I don't think so, Tott."

I was puzzled, "What do you mean?"

She was frowning, and then her face cleared. "I think that was the morphine."

"Morphine?"

"Yes, you've been taking in morphine for the pain. You know that paravertebral nerve block procedure you had? It's that. Think about it. They wouldn't have taken you to a restaurant in a bus, would they? You are ill, in hospital, you've just had a serious operation on your lung." She took my hand and shook it and with a giggle said, "There's no way you would be touring around Redhill in a mini-bus like Jack Nicholson in 'One Flew Over The Cuckoo's Nest.' Would you? It was the morphine. That's what it does, gives you all sorts of hallucinations."

"Really?"

"Yes." Big smile. "Really."

"Oh... okay."

I found it hard to believe the evening was an illusion. It had seemed so tangible, so physical. In a way, I was disappointed that it hadn't happened. Later, I realised Heather was right. After they had both gone and I was settling down, a couple of large dogs came dashing through the ward and past the bed. Another illusion. Like the big black flies, I had been swotting.

Morphine.

CHAPTER EIGHTEEN

Religiousity

A doctor came to see me. Tall, Asian. "Call me Mo," he instructed. Short for Mohammed, I decided. He had a friendly and likeable personality. He asked me several questions like those asked by the 'welfare' nurse yesterday. Who do I live with? Are there stairs in the house, how many? Etcetera. In a way it's comforting to know the NHS will still be concerned about me even when I have been discharged. Later, the welfare nurse came back and took me to a room where a set of stairs were set up and instructed me to climb up and down them a couple of times while she watched. A test I think I passed with colours flying.

H and C visited. After I point out to them both the ceiling is moving down towards us, Heather decides to have a word with Mo about the dosage of morphine I am taking in. Good idea. I saw several dogs of various sizes last night, running around as if Godstone Ward is their local park. I was tempted to ask her to see if, while he's at it, Mo could do something about RN who was also predominant last night with his repeated utterance of, "I pray to you God!" (a plea, by the way, God appears to be ignoring.) But I didn't as I reckon the doctor has enough on his plate without getting tangled up with religious nut cases. I think it would be easier to borrow a gun from somebody and shoot him.

MONDAY 8TH JULY

No dogs roaming the ward for the last couple of nights, and—joy of joys—the religious man seems to have forsaken his God as there has been a blissful silence from that direction. Long may it continue.

I have concluded being confined to hospital has compensations. I listened to an absorbing programme on the radio this afternoon all about the poem 'Adlestrop' by Edward Thomas. A poem, to my shame, I have never heard before. I blame that on the poor education dished out in the 1950s by East Suffolk County Council and the 1944 education act which at the age of eleven divided children into bright (those who would have the opportunity to go to a Grammar School and possibly University and the not-so-bright who would go to Secondary Modern School and leave at fifteen without any qualifications. The category I was condemned to.)

'Adelstrop invokes Englishness as we all imagine—or want—it to be, or how we think it used to be. Very English, anyway. The poem was written after the poet experienced a brief halt there in a train on 24th June 1914. I know. I've looked it up!

Anyway, I'll read it, 'Adlestrop' by Edward Thomas,

Yes, I remember Adlestrop—
The name, because one afternoon
Of heat the express train drew up there
Unwontedly. It was late June.

The steam hissed. Someone cleared his throat.
No one left and no one came
On the bare platform. What I saw
Was Adlestrop – only the name

And willows, willow herb, and grass,
And meadowsweet, and haycocks dry,
No whit less still and lonely fair
Than the high cloudlets in the sky.

And for that minute a blackbird sang
Close by, and round him, mistier
Farther and farther all the birds
Of Oxfordshire and Gloucestershire.

Adlestrop station is in Gloucestershire, and the only thing left after that Butcher Beeching closed it is the station sign re-sighted in a bus shelter.

Apart from listening to the radio, I laze here in bed watching hospital life circulate around me: the nurses tripping back and forwards, taking blood pressures, temperatures, and other measurements of the body behind round-the-bed blue curtains. Cleaners mopping, dusting, spraying, and wiping. Tea-trolleys rattling past, food distributed, doctors' visits. I can spend time reading, always an agreeable pastime, or get the laptop out and write, although I haven't accomplished too much of that this last week—but never mind, plenty of time. Except that phrase in my case, isn't as true as it was, is it? Cancer certainly concentrates the mind on your own mortality. And time takes on an entirely different characteristic. It seems to be accelerating just when I want it to slow down. If I believed in God, I would suspect he had given the earth a kick to speed up its progress around the sun just to exasperate me.

But it's quite agreeable to lay here and do nothing but think, and I find it astonishing the thoughts that travel through my head. They just float in unsystematically without my attempting to control them. Many of them are connected to the past. I think that's due to my present circumstance. When you know there is not a lot to look forward to it's only natural, I think, to look back. Or maybe it is simply my age. Old people are always dragging up the past, reminiscing. Boring their listeners to death. A few minutes ago, I was thinking about my mum.

I came home from school one day in February 1952, and she told me her mother had died and she had to go to Manchester for the funeral and would I accompany her? The next day, we were on a George Ewer Grey/Green coach on our way to London, Victoria. From there on another cold and draughty coach to Manchester.

My first visit to the city did not impress me. It was damp, cold, foggy, dirty, and the centre seemed to consist of a few car parks made out of old bombsites. While there, for the first time I met Mum's brothers and sisters: Jim, Henry, his wife Mona and elder sister Jessie.

The body was laid out in a coffin in the front room (the "parlour.") Each time I passed through, I averted my eyes not wanting to see a dead body. Before the Hearst arrived, Uncle Henry asked me "Do you want to see your Gran Chuck, before they take her away?" An invitation I declined as it didn't seem right to be viewing her for the first time in death.

The funeral started from the family home in Napier Street, Ardwick, concluding at Southern Cemetery to the south of the city. This was the first funeral I had attended and recall asking Uncle Jim a question about the grave. He answered by telling me it was a "double", meaning his mother had been buried on top of his father who had died some years previously. He concluded with a chuckle and said, "Oh aye, it's cheaper that way!"

After the funeral and back at Napier Street, I noticed a distinct change in the atmosphere within the family. It was only later, on the way home, Mum told me some friction had been created because Uncle Henry had married Mona the day before the funeral. It was his second marriage, and Jim, Jessie and Mum did not approve. "Fancy getting married the day before burying your mother!" Mum exclaimed, disgust and disapproval in her voice.

The evening of the funeral, Mum gave me half a crown saying, "Can you look after yourself this evening, pet lamb? "We are all going out for a drink, and we'll see you back here at eleven o'clock."

I went into the town centre and took a couple of rides on trolley buses. I liked the fast acceleration, the clicks and humming sound they made, but I didn't find them as good or satisfying as the Leicester trams I had spent so much time on during the war. I wandered through Piccadilly Gardens, and down Market Street and enjoyed looking at the lit advertising hoardings and the moving news displays outside the News Theatres. Now the war was over and there was no 'blackout,' the city centres were brightly lit with moving fluorescent adverts. A novelty to my eyes at that time. I wandered down Market Street and into one of the Lyons Corner Houses for a coffee and snack. While sitting there I remembered Mum had told us several time she had worked as a 'nippy' for Lyons in the 1920s, and it was there she had met dad. The result being her marriage to him and the production of four children, an unhappy divorce, and her return to Manchester.

Neither coach we travelled on overnight back to Felixstowe had heaters, and it was one of the coldest nights I have experienced— despite the blanket issued to each passenger as we boarded. It was one of the most uncomfortable and chilliest few hours I have ever had to endure.

* * *

A nurse interrupts my thoughts to take my blood pressure and temperature. She hardly speaks. The staff here are not like those in Copthorne Ward, where I was last year. In the weeks I was there, I got to know all the staff's names, Helen, Mathew, Isabel, Kunju, Shivani, and also the other patients, Darren, John, who died a couple of days after arriving in the ward, and Matt, who was involved in an accident that crippled him for life and killed two teenage girls. Andrew, the old boy opposite me who was constantly losing his alarm and forever shouting, "Nurse! Nurse!" Here I don't know any names of staff or patients. This is my fault as much as theirs. I should try, walk around, and start conversations like I did in Copthorne. Here it hasn't been so easy—or maybe I've been too wrapped up in my own troubles, or perhaps it's just that I can't be bothered. A thought and phrase that seems to pop into my head quite often these days, or is that me being too self-critical?

The nurse completes her checks on me, and I return to my thoughts.

After I left the BAA I started a video business—weddings, family events, instructional videos—all sorts of stuff. I was able to get work from Gatwick and Heathrow and Stansted because of my airport connections. When Cyril joined us, we called ourselves GHC Video Productions and both Cyril and Heather assisted me particularly so with the weddings. We used three cameras for those which gave us heaps of footage and were able to edit it into a decent wedding day video. Heather would interview some of the guests on camera, have you enjoyed the day? Do you want to give the couple a message? And similar. She was good at that.

After several years, we gave it up. It was, frankly, hard work, particularly weddings. They would often mean starting early in the morning and not finish 'til late at night, and it took me a further week to edit, add music, insert credits, etcetera, and complete it. I think both C and H were relieved when I decided to call it a day. Three cameras with three people, eight hours filming, and all for around £800. It just wasn't worth it.

GHC Video Production was successful, but it could have been much more successful. I lacked confidence. I think. I should have borrowed money and invested more into the business. These days, I imagine a good camera mounted on a drone would be part of the required equipment when shooting, though the stuff we had was up to date and produced a good product for the time.

CHAPTER NINETEEN

Home

FRIDAY 12ᵀᴴ JULY 2019

I get my things together after lunch is served, dress for the journey, and sit in the chair and wait for C and H. They arrive in the afternoon. We sit talking, waiting for someone to bring the discharge papers, and as we do, I start to notice discomfort in my stomach, it's gurgling, a slight pain. Heather notices.

"Are you all right, Tott?" She asks.

I shake my head and stand, point to the nearby toilet. "Gotta go." I mumbled and made my way to it. I got there a fraction late.

I'm getting really pissed off with this. The last couple of years has been one hurdle after another: there seems to be an obstacle to overcome every few hours—hospital visits, medical appointments to keep, a lobectomy, other surgery, also I now find I can no longer run for more than 50 yards without practically collapsing in a heap or no longer walk a mile without having to take a rest.

To think, and it doesn't seem so long ago, that I would cycle to work, ten miles from where we lived in Manchester. After work cycle to my girlfriend's house in higher Crumpsall, a further four miles and many evening we would walk to and around Heaton Park, then I would cycle home, another 14 miles. I kept that routine up for weeks. It worked out at around 28 miles a day, 140 miles a week. Each night, I would sink into bed and enjoy at least eight hours of uninterrupted sleep and never thought anything of it. Now, what have I got? Things like this happen, and eight hours uninterrupted sleep is a thing of the past. And I'm so slow these days, I view walking into town as an achievement. I still cycle, but my present bike is an e-bike; it is electrically assisted so climbing hills is a doddle. I can't get used to no longer being fit and worrying about my health. It's another consequence of getting old, and I'm getting sick of it.

I know, I've got to stop thinking negatively. Be more Heather-like and look on the bright side; be positive.

There's a knock on the door interrupting my thoughts. C asking if I'm okay as I've been in here a while now. I ask him to bring me some clean clothes.

All the necessary paperwork has been brought, and we are almost ready to go. As instructed, we sit in the nurse's area while they bring the various medicines, potions and pills I will need to continue my progress to the restoration of better health. When we get home, Heather carefully checks the various medicines and potions against the list given to her only to find one of them missing. She drove back to East Surrey to recover it.

-2021-

In early December of 2021, I developed all the indications of Covid 19—headaches, flu symptoms, sore throat, and feeling ill. We went to Uckfield Station where a Covid test centre had been set up in the car park. We asked the woman who attended me if Heather and Cyril could also take the test, but when she questioned them and discovered they did not have the symptoms required, she refused.

We should have insisted. How I wish we had.

My test proved positive, and the next day feeling quite under the weather, I crawled into bed. On the 12th of January, Heather wasn't feeling so good and stayed in bed, a most unusual event, as she would rarely admit to not feeling well; she didn't like being fussed over and would always resist it. The only time in our near sixty years together I can recall her succumbing to help was when she had hip problems and over a period of a couple of years both were replaced. After a few months, the first replacement became infected (the surgery had been carried out in a private hospital under the auspices of the NHS.) Returning from a visit to her cousin Pam one day in much pain, she was rushed into East Surry Hospital where she recovered after a fortnight.

When the pandemic struck us, Heather was in the front bedroom, and I in the small bedroom at the back. Cyril was kept busy looking after us, up and down the stairs, bringing us cups of tea, snacks, medicines etcetera, answering shouted requests. Several times, I walked along the landing and looked in on her as she did me. Conversations were usually brief:

"How are you feeling, Bumble?"

"I'm okay, how about you?"

"Yeah, not too bad." Then she would urge me to leave her alone and return to my bedroom.

On the 14th of January at about seven in the morning, I was awake and listening to the news on the radio when I heard a loud bang. Something had fallen. I got up and went to Heather's room. She was on the floor, between the bedroom and her ensuite bathroom, barely conscious. I managed to get her into a sitting position with her back leaning against the wall. She looked woozy and stared at me without saying anything. I'm not confident she was seeing me. I tried to lift her further but couldn't. I called Cyril thinking between us we could get her back into bed, and although we struggled, it proved to be impossible. She was a dead weight, semi-conscious, and we were both nervous about making things worse. We called an ambulance. It arrived quickly and the two medics—one male, one female—were able to get her back into bed and comfortable. They took her temperature, blood pressure, and checked her over. By now, she was conscious, talking and seemed to be okay. The medics advised us to have her checked for Covid and left. We obtained a test kit and sent it off.

For the next few days, we continued to visit each other. She seemed okay, if less chatty than usual, and I could tell she wasn't getting over the wretched virus as I seemed to be. By now, I was feeling okay and decided to dress and join Cyril downstairs, but before going down, I looked in on her. She was sitting up and leaning against the headboard, fast asleep. I didn't attempt to wake her, thinking sleep was a good thing. I joined Cyril in the TV room. At about ten o'clock, I looked in on Heather to say 'goodnight'. She was in the same position as she had been earlier, against the headboard, asleep.

"Going to bed now, Bumble." I said. She didn't answer, still asleep. I walked over and touched her bare arm. It was stone cold, and now I could see she wasn't breathing. I called Cyril, dialled 999. The woman who answered asked, "Is she breathing?" Have you administered CPR? The answer was 'no' to each. Under her direction, we eased Heather off the bed and Cyril administered CPR. I couldn't believe this was happening. She was on the floor, inert, no sign of life. It was too late. Heather had gone. We couldn't get her back. Cyril and I were shocked beyond words. We couldn't believe our happy, smiling-so-alive Heather had died. I was devastated. Cyril and I were both devastated. Heather was the centre of our lives. The three of us were completely and utterly happy together. It was so cruel, such a shock. We had our 54th wedding anniversary in September and had known each other for much longer. I'll never get used to being without her. That awful evening plays over and over in my head, and I question myself again and again. Why didn't I call in to check on her again while we were watching television that evening? Why didn't we *insist* on her having a Covid test? I should have urged—demanded—the two medics who came to the house on the 14th of January had taken her to hospital for a thorough check.

A policeman came to the door, probably because of the 999 call. He took details, ordered an ambulance, and Heather was taken to Worthing Coroner's Office where, I assumed she would be subjected to a post-mortem. This wasn't the case. It was some time before a death certificate was issued. Delays, and any change to routine during this period was always blamed on the pandemic. We were not able to arrange the funeral until a month had passed. For some reason, the coroner's office sent the details of Heather's passing to our local GP, and it was he who decided her demise was due to Covid 19. I spoke to him, making it clear I wasn't convinced it was the pandemic responsible. She hadn't seen the doctor for months and he gave me a politician's answer, lots of words but saying nothing palpable.

I was and am still sure there was more to it than that. This was at the time when if you were run over by a bus and had recently tested for Covid—Covid would be blamed for your death. She had collapsed several days before and the two medics who attended had checked her over, taking her blood pressure, temperature, etc., and found nothing wrong, merely advising us to have her tested for Covid, and although the test had been sent off, we never received a reply. Her dad had died because of a heart problem, and I believe it ran in the family. Could it have been that? I'll never know now.

Because of the pandemic rules prevalent at the time, only 30 people were allowed to be at her funeral. There would have been many more had this restriction not been in existence at the time.

To borrow from the late Queen's view of 1992, 2021 has been my "annus horribiles". The death of Heather, and less than six months later being told I have lung cancer, how could things be worse?

For a while, it seemed like too much to bear. At the time had there been a 'painless permanent sleep' pill on the market I would have taken it.

CHAPTER TWENTY

Conclusion(s)

FRIDAY 13ᵗʰ JULY

I t's six months since I was told I had lung cancer. Stage 4 Incurable. Eighteen months since Heather died. Her sudden death brought me despair, depression, and the stark reality of loss. Heather had seen me through colon cancer in 2019 with her positive cheerfulness despite the negativity that surrounds the disease; she had kept me out of depression with her smiling jollity and upbeat attitude to life, so that now, without her, depression, and negative thoughts creep in despite my efforts to resist them. Heather's not here so there is an emptiness in my life, an awful gap, a persistent feeling of self-reproach, sorrow, remorse, and above all guilt. Guilt over the wrongs I did her over the years. Regretfully, there were many. So many, I won't attempt to list them. She is in my head from the moment I wake, from what these days is a poor night's sleep, to the time I fall asleep again thoughts of her dance around in my head. It's a daily torment. Sleep is a great escape and I turn to it often.

I know that I am still in mourning. I am unable to talk about Heather without a lump forming in my throat and tears appearing in my eyes to the awkwardness of myself and the embarrassment of those I'm with.

But there is one good thing that has come out of all this, and here I'm doing a 'Heather' and looking on the bright side. Being positive.

My brother Cyril.

He has been such a strong and reliable support. I know the loss of Heather has affected him almost as much as it has affected me, and yet he has watched over me, making sure I stay sane and don't do anything silly; he tries to cheer me up when I get down and makes daft remarks every now and then that cause me to laugh. He does more than his share of running the house, cooks, helps with the garden, keeps a very sharp eye on our income; has organised a couple of holidays; he always comes with me when I attend hospital for the various checks and tests I have. We seldom argue, and when we do it is always light-hearted and usually concerned with the present Tory government—the worst I have ever known. They seem to be hellbent on making sure the rich get richer, and we at the other end of the scale, poorer. The shameful thing is they are succeeding, and the worst thing is they seem to be slowly, covertly, stealthily, and sneakily reducing the NHS to a shadow of its former self.

Recently, Cyril seems to have taken over Heather's persona. He keeps telling me he believes East Sussex Hospital, Mr Smith, Mr Aslam. Dr Nimako have all got it wrong. It's a mistake. I haven't got lung cancer at all. He refers me to the 8th of August 2018 when we went to East Surrey Hospital to hear the verdict after the early tests and Neil Smith said, *"Well, Mr Thornhill, we have had a report of the CAT-scan that you had on your chest, there was a place that we thought might be a problem, but we are assured by the chest experts that it's nothing, so…that's good enough for me."* Since that date, nothing seems to have altered. I read about people who have cancer and are bravely fighting it. I'm not bravely fighting it. I'm just living with the notion of it. And, frankly, on my day-to-day routine, I don't notice anything to 'live with'. I have no pain. This "awful crippling and painful disease" as I have seen it described, doesn't seem to be associated with me. I am living life as I always have. Getting up in the morning, reading, watching television, riding the bike, going for a drink, sitting at the computer, writing, socialising with friends. The worst part of all this, I think, is how it is affecting me mentally.

* * *

These last few weeks I have ceased to worry about death. I know it's coming, and it won't be too far into the future. My 86th birthday is close now, so my final departure could easily be any day, any time. I don't feel ill; in fact, some days I feel very well. My brain is still working *(Are you alert, Tott? Heather would say to me. Yes, Bumble, I'm chief Lert.)*

However, putting the cancer aside for a moment, it is becoming clear to me that my demise is just as likely to be because of the ageing process. I hope that is the case. The cancer, if indeed I *do* have it is still not affecting me, apart from the mental turmoil it creates. If it is to be the cancer that finishes me, I fear what might accompany it—pain, loss of control, and other discomforts which can come with this disease as the grim reaper takes charge. Heather went to sleep and didn't wake up. I hope that happens to me. It is less traumatic for all concerned. Heather didn't have any pain, so far as I know. I do hope she didn't. If she did surely, she would have called us on her mobile? And then we would have been with her when the end came, instead of downstairs watching television, and we may have been able to save her. But neither of us had the slightest inkling she was as ill as she clearly was. This is the kind of thought that tumbles through my mind all the time, never stops. For a while I imagined I *might* go off the rails, become 'a little disturbed,' as they say. But that hasn't happened; well, I don't think it has. I suspect I am more likely to become a victim of dementia; my short-term memory seems to be getting worse, I keep leaving the tap in the kitchen on, forgetting names of people and words I shouldn't forget, put things down and then unable to find where I put them, that kind of thing. But time will tell, I suppose. I am assured these things happen when you are well into your eighties.

So, my fear of death is becoming less, it no longer dominates my thoughts. What has taken its place is the fear that Cyril may die before me. I am very aware that is a possibility. He is 80 in December. Has type 2 diabetes and takes several pills every day to control it. I am nervous about him exiting before me for I know, if he does go, I will be lost. Apart from the support he gives, the control of our income, help around the house, cooking, and shopping, we actively enjoy each other's company. So the fear of losing him is… well, a little selfish perhaps. Such a loss, to me, would be almost as devastating as the loss of Heather. Not quite that bad, of course, but not too far off it.

The first few days after Heather died, I wanted to join her, thinking *If I died too, we would be together again.* Like my dad who must have had similar thoughts for on his memorial stone that Richard and Derek took us to see in July 2021 it says 'Betty Thornhill, died 10.11.80 aged 64'. *(That was no age at all! Dad must have gone through what I've been going through these last couple of years.)* It also says: D.O. "Dickie" Thornhill *reunited* 5.10.89. So, he believed they would be together again. But the thoughts of me joining Heather didn't last. I'm not spiritual as I think this narrative has made clear. But lately, I keep imagining Heather is watching me, and I find myself talking to her; especially so when I'm on my own in the garden, or the greenhouse (which we bought for her, and she spent a lot of time in.) "Hello, Bumble," I say. "How are you today? I'm here again, trying to make the garden nice for you, putting in plenty of flowers. I know how you loved them." I tell myself it's silly, but I do it anyway. It's a little like the non-believer who prays. (Just in case there is a God who cares and listens, even though underneath it all he knows there isn't, and nobody is listening.)

If Cyril does die first, (we have talked about this), I think I would investigate getting myself into one of these places where you buy a flat set-in attractive grounds, and the company looks after all the maintenance. They usually have a club room and bar and other amenities so you can always find some companionship. We went to look at one just outside Horsham about three years ago, but when we got there to inspect, Heather, who had not been keen from the start, balked and refused to get out of the car and inspect the place.

I thought it was a good idea at the time, but Heather didn't so that was that. *I'm sorry I put you through that, Bumble.*

Anyway, I dropped the idea and didn't attempt to look at any similar facilities. I don't think Cyril was keen either, so it was probably just as well. He kept mentioning the quarterly maintenance costs, "Which will keep going up."

Things are very different now, but I have urged him to think again when I've gone, though when I've gone, and he sold the house he would be able to afford it easily, unless there is a collapse in the housing market and the way the cost of living is rising right now, and inflation is hitting us I wouldn't be surprised. He talks of moving back up north if he is left on his own. I don't have confidence in that idea either. As things are he worries about Lindsay and Stephen. Being geographically closer to them would, I think, cause him to become more involved with their everyday lives and each problem that came their way would create more possibilities for him to worry. But who knows what will happen? We always assumed Uncle Jim, who lived with Mum, would die before her, but he lived for several years after Mum passed away.

I am now in my 87th year, and as I have previously mentioned, during these last couple of years I have slowed down a great deal both mentally and physically; I walk much more slowly, I don't sleep as well as I once did, I forget words, forget names, am easily confused, in fact I recently life has become difficult to navigate.

I do not recommend old age.

I am beginning to understand why very old people look forward to death, something I have never previously understood. Don't misunderstand, I rush to add, I am not yet in that frame of mind, and while Cyril is with me, I don't think I will be.

Retirement has been good, this I do recommend, for it means being free of the petty disciplines and control of an employer. It's how life should be when you are young. Retirement is freedom. Within reason you can say do and go where you want. But best of all is the inheritance of time. Time to pursue new interests, travel, visit friends, write, read, reflect.

My childhood had happy moments. Mum would often sing us to sleep, and in those days, she was very loving. My elder brother, Roy, younger brother Cyril, and sister Stephanie would often accuse me of being Mum's 'favourite', an accusation I would deny. But truth to tell, they were right. I was. Also, in those days at bedtime Roy would tell me stories—he had a terrific imagination. Roy also bullied me, which created hours of wretchedness. The 1940s brought us the excitement of the war and Roy and me watching the Bristol blitz through the bedroom window of "Lingerfield' the house in Brentry, the small hamlet where we lived during the early 40s. The 1950s were a miserable time. Rationing, shortages, queues, bombsites, National Service, the cold war, Mum's divorce, our move to Manchester. With the 1960s a slow improvement came to my life and to Britain in general. It was less restrictive, London was 'swinging,' the BBC lost its monopoly, the pirate radio stations gave us all day pop records, I had my first love affair that brought me much joy and an equal amount of misery.

There is no doubt in my mind the very best years have been from the seventies until now (I except the devastation of 2021 from this).

I am close to the end now. The end of this short book, I mean. The end of my life, too, of course. A few random thoughts to leave you with. Has it been a good life? Difficult to decide— it's the only one I have any experience of so far. But I do know the years from 2000 to 2020 were my happiest. My teens and early twenties were not good. 2021 was the very worst and unhappiest. The best thing that has happened to me? Meeting and marrying Heather, the worst? Starting to smoke. How foolish that was. Readers, don't fall into the same trap and become a slave to the tobacco companies. One other thing, if I may: Get yourself checked. At the very least have a blood test.

Finally, before I leave you, I should mention this thought that keeps creeping back. And I know this isn't possible, at the least it's extremely unlikely, and there is absolutely no evidence for it, but I cling on to the idea:-Perhaps...maybe... I *will* see Heather again. And she will say, "Don't worry, Totty, I've forgiven you." And she'll put her arms around me, and we will dance around the kitchen as I hum The Cuckoo Waltz. Wouldn't that be wonderful?

East Grinstead, June 2023
Gerryhugh76@gmail.com

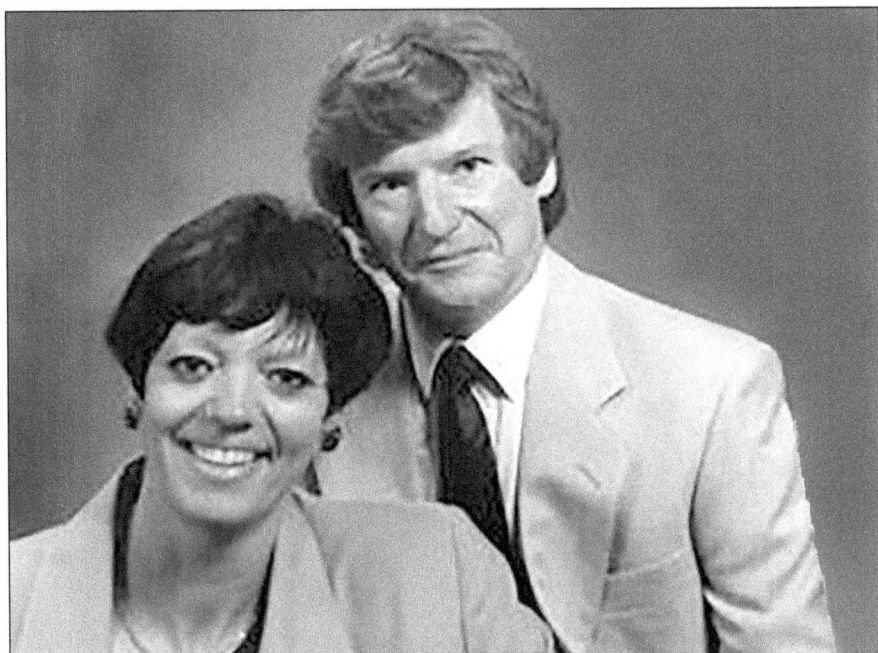

The author with late wife, Heather

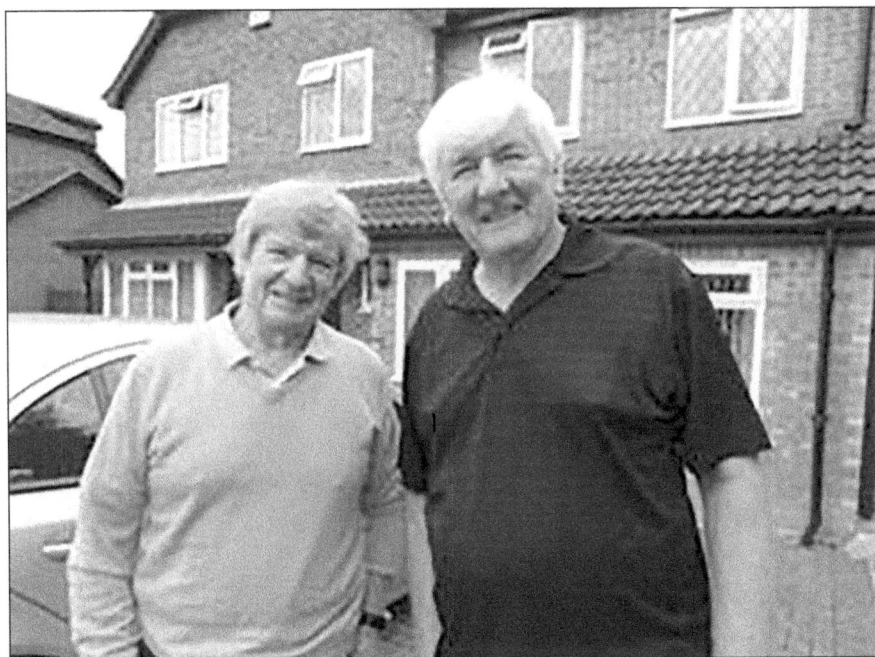

With brother Cyril

Milton Keynes UK
Ingram Content Group UK Ltd.
UKHW012149131223
434335UK00002B/16

9 781959 224808